THE COMPLETE* GUIDE TO TRANSFORMING THE PATIENT EXPERIENCE

*JUST ADD YOUR TALENT, PASSION, AND HARD WORK.

GARY ADAMSON AND SONIA RHODES

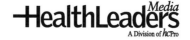

HealthLeaders *Media*
A Division of *hc*Pro

Gary Adamson, Author
Sonia Rhodes, Author
Gienna Shaw, Senior Editor
Amy Anthony, Executive Editor
Matt Cann, Group Publisher
Doug Ponte, Cover Designer

Janell Lukac, Graphic Artist
Audrey Doyle, Copyeditor
Amy Cohen, Proofreader
Matt Sharpe, Production Supervisor
Susan Darbyshire, Art Director
Jean St. Pierre, Director of Operations

Advice given is general. Readers should consult professional counsel for specific legal, ethical, or clinical questions. Arrangements can be made for quantity discounts. For more information, contact:

HCPro, Inc.
P.O. Box 1168
Marblehead, MA 01945
Telephone: 800/650-6787 or 781/639-1872
Fax: 781/639-2982
E-mail: *customerservice@hcpro.com*

HCPro, Inc., is the parent company of HealthLeaders Media.
Visit HCPro at its World Wide Web sites:
www.healthleadersmedia.com, www.hcpro.com, and *www.hcmarketplace.com*

10/2009
21729

Contents

Contents

The Complete Guide to Transforming the Patient Experience

About the Authors

Gary Adamson

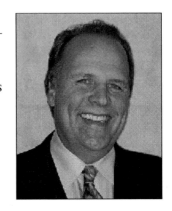

Gary Adamson is the chief experience officer of Starizon Studio, an experience design and staging firm. Adamson's work at Starizon is just the latest chapter in a career dedicated to expanding the boundaries of what's possible. He began his career in 1978 as vice president of Swedish Health Systems in Denver, where he started the nation's first and most comprehensive hospital-based wellness program and consulted with hundreds of hospitals on how to build healthier communities.

In 1983, Adamson began a new business venture, Unison Marketing and Communications, one of the first national marketing firms to be focused solely on healthcare. He worked in every part of the country with health systems, hospitals, foundations, medical groups, health plans, healthcare associations, and a wide variety of health-related businesses to develop unified innovations in strategy, operations, and communications. In 1993, he merged Unison with Medimetrix, a national managed care consulting company, and the combined firm went on to be a rare, two-time Inc. 500 Fastest Growing Private Company in the United States.

Through this work, Adamson consistently found a detrimental gap between the brand promise that organizations made and the brand experience they delivered.

Given this, he set out to find the most innovative thinking and best people to help solve this complex business challenge. From this, Starizon was born. In 1999, he cofounded Starizon with the purpose of helping organizations intentionally design the experiences that would significantly transform them and strengthen their brand success. To that end, he created the proprietary 6-I's of Experience® process, which is critical to the exploration and discovery employed with Starizon members. Clients have included companies in a wide variety of sizes and industries from start-ups to Microsoft, John Deere, Dell, The Miami Dolphins, The Methodist Hospital/Texas Medical Center, and Sharp Healthcare. Starizon was also recognized as an Inc. 500 Fastest Growing Private Company in 2005.

Adamson is a highly rated speaker at regional, national, and international conferences. He received his master's degree in health administration from the University of Colorado, to which he attributes much of his forward-thinking skills to the time he spent there with noted healthcare futurist Leland R. Kaiser. He received his undergraduate degree from the University of Notre Dame, to which he attributes his occasional mood swings during the football season.

Sonia Rhodes

Sonia Rhodes is the vice president of customer strategy, The Sharp Experience & The Sharp University for Sharp HealthCare, a nonprofit integrated healthcare delivery system, and San Diego's largest private employer. Rhodes leads The Sharp Experience—an organizational performance improvement initiative designed to transform the

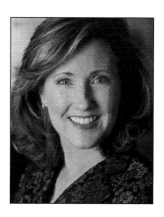

healthcare experience for staff, physicians, and customers. Her passion to make the healthcare experience the best it can be is evidenced in all that she does.

As a result of this focused organizational improvement effort, Sharp HealthCare was one of five organizations awarded the 2007 Malcolm Baldrige National Quality Award—the nation's highest presidential honor for quality and organizational performance excellence—by President George W. Bush and Commerce Secretary Carlos Gutierrez.

In addition to The Sharp Experience, Rhodes also conceptualized, launched, and actively directs The Sharp University, a corporate university focused on the education and development of over 1,400 Sharp leaders and nearly 14,000 Sharp associates.

Rhodes also provides oversight and leadership for Sharp's overarching customer strategy, marketing technologies, and research endeavors, including Web strategy and design, customer contact centers, 24-hour nurse advice service, and consumer research. With more than 15 years at Sharp HealthCare and more than 20 years in the healthcare industry, she is a frequent national speaker on creating better healthcare experiences.

In 2005, Rhodes was one of the first in the nation to be recognized for her individual achievement in the emerging Experience Economy, receiving the Experience Management Achievement (EMA) award. She holds a bachelor's degree from the University of California and Santa Barbara in health education and sociology.

Acknowledgments

Gary Adamson

I dedicate this book to all the inspiring moments in my life when my wife, my kids, my parents, my teachers, my partners, my employees, my clients, as well as unknown strangers and famous explorers lived this idea:

> *Be willing, at any moment, to sacrifice all that you are, for all that you could become.*
>
> —*Maharishi Mahesh Yogi*

It is in these bold and hope-filled actions where I learned that changing the world is not only possible, it is why we are here. Carpe Diem.

Sonia Rhodes

With immense gratitude to those who have gifted my life as mentors, colleagues, provocateurs, and friends, thank you for sharing your spark of possibility with me and for encouraging me to dream big and live that dream into existence. A special thank you to the people who have courageously shared their less-than-ideal healthcare experiences with me (especially my dad)—you are what this book and this work are all about.

Acknowledgments

To my incredible family, with love and appreciation for inspiring me every day to learn more, do more, and be more than I ever imagined. Your love and light illuminate each step of this journey and you serve as my daily reminder to do everything I can to make the world a better place.

This book would not be possible without the hard work and passionate commitment of the 14,000 team members of Sharp HealthCare—all dedicated to making the healthcare experience the best that it can be. Their vision, leadership, and heart-filled work have made it possible for me to share their story.

     The Complete Guide to Transforming the Patient Experience

Foreword

By B. Joseph Pine II

I still remember vividly that day in June 2002 when I stood in Aspire, an appropriately aspirational room in the still uncompleted yet already inspirational place called Starizon. I had come to Keystone, CO, to see what this place would be, what it could become; to understand the idea its founder, Gary Adamson, had for transforming companies into premier experience stagers; and to learn his "6-I's" approach for staging engaging experiences. And there he was, spouting my very own words back at me, reading out loud from (as he never tires of stating) page 193 of The Experience Economy:

> *Consider also the business-to-business example of management consulting, another industry that typically charges for the service activities workers perform, rather than for the actual transformation of clients. If consultants truly viewed themselves as being in the business of transformation, they would, like fitness centers, spend much more time in the up-front diagnosis phase, identifying clients' strategic needs as well as their capacity for change. They would stop writing analytical documents (the tangible goods of the present-day, PowerPoint-driven consulting industry) and start staging memorable events that would enable the client first to experience what it would be like to live and work in a world where the strategy has been achieved and then to actually create that future world. (While, of course, providing appropriate memorabilia for each experience that would be very different from today's sterile binders.) Most important, they would follow*

through to ensure each client actually achieved its stated strategy, or else risk losing some or all of its fee. Wholly successful engagements, perhaps commemorated with appropriate emblems, would result in even greater revenue than that received today for mere services.

Gary told me those words inspired his creation of the very idea, the approach, and finally the place of Starizon—a new kind of management consulting company where explorers would indeed live and work in a place that had been designed with the very approach they were learning to apply to their own business, and where 25% of its fees would be at risk, completely dependent on the client's perception of the transformational value received. And he asked me to join him in this groundbreaking endeavor.

How could I refuse?

Although that was the beginning of our journey together, it was the culmination of a learning curve that began (I learned later) when Gary read the article "Welcome to the Experience Economy" that Jim Gilmore, my partner in the Cleveland-based Strategic Horizons, LLP, and I wrote for the July/August 1998 *Harvard Business Review.* He realized it explained a lot about what he was seeing in the healthcare industry—that the way out of the commoditization trap so many hospitals found themselves in was to create intentional, personal experiences for patients, family members, and even workers.

Gary had by that time sold the healthcare marketing agency that he and his wife, Leigh, had built up, Unison, to Medimetrix in Cleveland. The announcement mentioned that Unison was an expert in one-to-one marketing and mass customization, so unbeknownst to me, Scott Lash, one of my other SHLLP partners, saw the local notice and added Gary to our database. Shortly after reading the article and beginning to think that this experience stuff might very well lead to the next stage in his career, he received an invitation to the very first thinkAbout event that Jim and I staged in November 1998 in Cleveland. Our opportunity to practice what we preach, it was at that event—with my "intellectual idol" Stan Davis (the developer of the concept of Mass Customization) as our talent—where Jim and I fully segued from popularizers of that concept to progenitors of our very own Progression of Economic Value, which details the fundamental economic shifts from commodities, goods, and services to experiences and transformations. I can still remember how Stan's initial reaction was to argue against experiences and transformations as distinct economic offerings, and how Gary led the charge of the entire group in defending our ideas.

Since first being exposed to the ideas, Gary had put together a business plan (including the idea of creating a place) for Medimetrix to lead healthcare into the experience economy. His partners, however, were skeptical and unconvinced. Buoyed by his own beliefs and the energy he retained from thinkAbout, Gary left the company in January, 1999. Everyone thought he was crazy—oh, they could understand why experiences were important, but not why he needed to create his own place dedicated to the concept: Why in the world would clients want to travel to him, instead of the consultant to the client, as it had always been done? Or why he wanted to give every project a 25% haircut, for surely no client would ever pay a dime more than they had to.

But Gary shot up that learning curve, hunkering down to develop the "6-I's" approach to experience design, testing it out with clients—the first one being San Juan Regional Medical Center in Farmington, NM—and thinking about how he could in fact create that place. He came to our second thinkAbout event, held in Los Angeles in September 1999, and asked whether he could meet with me afterward. So at a local Jamba Juice, Gary talked of his approach and laid out his plans of creating a singular place in Keystone, called Starizon. And truth be told, my reaction was closer to his old partners at Medimetrix than to his future partner!

But Gary got plugging along that learning curve, buying just the right property, seeking investors, and creating architectural drawings. He even showed me his drawings at thinkAbout 2001 in Las Vegas (unable to participate in the previous year's event in Chicago, I met Leigh for the first time there), where I began to realize that he truly was serious—this place was being built! And that he was seriously onto something.

Less than a year later, I was standing in that place, listening to my words read back to me, and finding my head nodding at the question, "Do you want to be a part of the place you inspired?" In September 2002, Starizon opened its doors with Gary and me as partners.

Meanwhile, Sonia Rhodes took a very different journey to arrive at the same metaphorical place: the top of the Experience Economy learning curve as a driving force behind Sharp HealthCare receiving the Malcolm Baldrige National Quality Award in 2007. It was a family healthcare experience in the late 1990s that opened her eyes to the need for a dramatically different healthcare experience. She told me she studied and read everything she could get her hands on, but all of the typical customer service–oriented books out there were good, but not enough. They didn't get to the heart of the matter.

In late 1999, Sonia's husband just happened to attend a National Funeral Directors Association conference (well, not "just happened"—he does work for Batesville Casket), where some guy named Jim Gilmore was the keynote speaker, talking about something he called the experience economy. Sonia's husband brought home a copy of the video of the keynote presentation and told her this guy was talking about everything she'd been talking about. After watching the video and then finding and devouring our book, she told me her reaction was, "I'm not crazy!"

As debatable as that might be, Sonia came to our thinkAbout 2000 event in Chicago (and has come back to each one since then to recharge her batteries and continue to move up her own learning curve by discovering the best principles of the Experience Economy). This began a comprehensive, nationwide investigation into creating better employee and customer experiences, which Sonia and the Sharp team ultimately wove into the core of what became The Sharp Experience— her health system's organizationwide performance and experience improvement initiative launched in fall 2001.

It was at thinkAbout 2002 where Sonia and Gary really first got to know each other. We bought out Hotel Avante in Mountain View, CA, one of Chip Conley's Joie de Vivre Hospitality hotels (our 2001 Experience Stager of the Year, or EXPY, award winner). Taking a cue from the Pixar hit *Monsters*, we invented "brain-dorming" and asked every participant to post a description of his or her business and experience on his or her "dorm room" door. So Sonia, with her typical over-the-top enthusiasm, posted her fire-themed Sharp Experience initiative, while Gary (and Leigh), in typically inspirational language, posted pictures and a description of Starizon, which had opened that very month.

That following summer, Sonia invited me to present to 1,300 leaders at Sharp's quarterly leadership development session, and that fall to all 14,000 Sharp team members at its annual All-Staff Assembly sessions—a unique employee engagement experience designed to further The Sharp Experience endeavor. And the more I visited, the more I learned about Sharp's commitment to creating a unique healthcare experience. I visited Endoscopy and learned of its signature moment, inspired by visits to local five-star San Diego hotels. I found out about how Sharp patients received personal, handwritten thank-you notes from someone they touched during their visits. And I discovered that when something goes wrong at Sharp, their first reaction is not to circle the legal wagons and clam up, but to apologize, person to person.

It is no wonder that in September 2005, when Jim Gilmore and I created the Experience Management Award for our annual thinkAbout event, held that year not coincidentally in Keystone, the very first award ceremony jointly honored two people who, above all others, embraced the principles that we outlined in The Experience Economy and put them into practice: Gary Adamson and Sonia Rhodes.

To get to that point, they each had to follow steep learning curves, ones that began with a basic dissatisfaction of how things were and a deep commitment to how things could be. If you are dissatisfied with what passes for conventional wisdom in the healthcare industry and are committed to doing it differently, to being authentically different, there is no better way to begin your journey than to heed the lessons that Gary and Sonia lay out in this book. You have in your hands the best of all worlds: the approach of Starizon, the story of Sharp HealthCare, and the strength of your commitment.

B. Joseph Pine II is the cofounder of Strategic Horizons, LLP, and Principal Innovator at Starizon, Inc. He coauthored *The Experience Economy and Authenticity: What Consumers Really Want* with Jim Gilmore, and can be reached at 651/653-6850 or *bjp2@aol.com.*

THE STORY IN THE STONE:
The State of the Experience in Healthcare

Ask archeologists anywhere why they devote themselves to work that is both groundbreaking and backbreaking, and you will no doubt hear them talk about decoding the "story in the stone." Every dig tells the story of advancement, decline, and advancement again. From survival societies with crude tools and a single-minded focus on reacting to immediate danger to aspiring societies with higher thoughts of the future and the rudimentary beginnings of an organized approach to accomplished societies where intentionally designed and sophisticated systems create the desired future, the story told in each layer and between the layers is a fascinating one. And because progress is not a tidy, straight-line affair, what archaeologists uncover and plot in their work is nothing less than humankind's learning curve.

But you don't have to be an Indiana Jones–style adventurer or understand the intricacies of carbon dating to make similar discoveries in the learning curve of business. Because organizations are themselves small societies, you can see survival, aspiring, and accomplished versions there, too. Think of airlines before flight simulators, computer-assisted piloting, and Six Sigma safety systems. Consider automobiles before crash test dummies, on-board diagnostics/navigation, and alternative fuel use. In healthcare, remember quality before sterile technique, advanced diagnostics, minimally invasive procedures, evidence-based practices, and much stricter peer review.

A National Study to Unearth the Truth

Today there is an increasing amount of conversation about the patient experience in healthcare. But opinions vary widely. Healthcare executives describe patient experience as everything from a small personal touch to a huge cultural change. Some leaders embrace it as a "life's work" and others ignore it as an "unfunded distraction."

"Our intentional patient experience is the focus of everything we do. Our outcomes, because of it, have been amazing both in transformed lives and [in] financial results," one leader says. Another counters, "Patient experience is smoke and mirrors. Money and time drive the system, not quality of care."

So where are we, really? What is the truth when it comes to patient experience?

To answer these questions, HealthLeaders Media conducted a national benchmarking survey, asking top healthcare leaders to weigh in on their thoughts, beliefs, and ideas about patient experience. Conducted and published in October 2009, the study goes beyond the typical review of "best practices" and patient satisfaction to utilize instruments and insights based on the "best principles" of successful experience stagers, both inside and outside of healthcare. It is nothing less than an "archeological dig" that seeks to uncover the level of current practice (survival, aspiring, or accomplished), and speed progress on a learning curve vital to healthcare's future success.

The following is some of what was unearthed.

Patient experience a top priority

Healthcare institutions are realizing the growing importance of patient experience. And they are realizing it in a big way. Nearly 90% of senior healthcare leaders said patient experience is one of their top five priorities. And the figure jumps even higher when asked about their priorities five years from now.

A surprising 55% report that the patient experience is a major consideration in all decisions, whereas only 6% report that decisions are not reached through a patient experience lens. Seventy-four percent of respondents agreed with the statement "Patient experience drives demand for care just as strongly as clinical quality does," and interestingly, one of the six people who strongly disagreed with the statement did so because of the belief that "Patient experience drives demand for care much more strongly than clinical quality does."

The story in the stone: Healthcare has gone beyond a survival society to an aspiring society when it comes to patient experience.

Management responses lagging

However, much of the data collected suggest major disconnects between healthcare leaders' stated priority of patient experience and the management direction, accountability, and structure they provide in its pursuit.

Fifty-nine percent of respondents said their organization has not done a strong job of establishing "a defined mission and strategy that guides the work of all employees" when it comes to patient experience. The number one response (24.5%) to the question of who owns responsibility for the patient experience was "the CEO." The number two answer (20.5%) was "no one specific individual." Only 1% of respondents said they have a chief experience officer or similar title. The wide variety of responses among those who answered "other" shows an ill-defined response to this new management priority and mentality. More than one-third of the respondents said there is "significant room for improvement" in the way their organization operationally connects the patient experience function across all departments.

The story in the stone: Patient experience is a high priority plagued by low organizational direction.

Innovation inward-focused

Considering the low marks healthcare continues to receive relative to other industries in the rating of its customer experience, it would be reasonable to expect a good deal of study of outside industries to help accelerate innovation. This was not the case. Most respondents (62%) reported that they observe other organizations in

The Complete Guide to Transforming the Patient Experience

healthcare to generate their own patient experience ideas—meaning that healthcare is by and large a self-referencing industry, relying on borrowed innovations. Another 63% of respondents reported that they only "occasionally" seek professional outside strategy counsel for help in generating patient experience innovations. And yet only 31% of respondents rated themselves as innovating "often" in this new area. Healthcare would do well to heed Albert Einstein's advice that "the problems of this world will not be solved by the same level of thinking that created them."

The story in the stone: Patient experience is a high priority stalled by low innovation.

Technology falls short

Perhaps as a result of the lack of innovative practices, the majority of respondents, 69%, rated their use of technology to remember personal details about patients (beyond medical and demographic information) as "fair" or "poor." Given that meaningful experiences are inherently personal and that staging them successfully requires the ability to orchestrate and anticipate and not just react, this technologic shortcoming will doom many efforts from the outset. Although huge investments are being made in IT, much of it is being spent to automate the old instead of enable the new.

The story in the stone: Patient experience is a high priority stymied by low technological support.

Facilities unsupportive

Despite the national trend toward the design and construction of "healing environments," 45% of the respondents rated the design of their facility as "fair" or "poor" in its ability to support an outstanding patient experience. Maybe it's the heritage of semiprivate rooms, or the history of sterile, uninviting functional space, or the lack of designated "onstage" and "offstage" areas. Whatever it is, even the best of patient experience intentions is too often being thwarted by the surroundings in which they are performed.

The story in the stone: Patient experience is a high priority with low translation into the physical environment.

Financial support lacking

This tells much about the real priority of patient experience initiatives. The most oft-cited stumbling block to adopting or enhancing a patient experience strategy was "lack of funding or budgeting priority." Seventy-six percent of organizations have a budget of less than $100,000 (46% are spending less than $50,000). How frequently does a real top-five priority fail to garner meaningful funds during the budgetary cycle? Part of the problem may be that expenditures for patient experience are doled out into a wide variety of small, unrelated categories, effectively obscuring the size of the overall commitment. One thing is for sure, however: Healthcare leaders know they are damaging their own credibility and that of their patient experience intentions by lending verbal but not monetary support.

The story in the stone: Patient experience is stated as a high priority, but the claim has low credibility because of budgetary practices.

  The Complete Guide to Transforming the Patient Experience

Employee training and development increased

Many institutions understand that employees carry much of the patient experience responsibility. Eighty-five percent either currently have or are about to launch employee training and development programs with an increased focus on patient experience. This is the closest thing to a universal institutional response seen in the survey. Fifty-eight percent also report the use of employee reward and recognition programs to support patient experience improvement. Few, however, pointed to the design of an intentional employee experience as an important precursor for the staging of an intentional patient experience. And with all the disconnects in definition and approach documented throughout the rest of the study, it brings into question the effectiveness of all that training.

The story in the stone: Patient experience is a high priority with an increasingly important focus on employee development.

Definition indistinct

Perhaps an explanation for the shortage of innovative and comprehensive responses to patient experience is the lack of distinction between patient satisfaction and patient experience.

Patient experience is described using standard terms instead of embracing a new definition. More than half (57%) of respondents describe it as "patient-centered care" or "exceptional customer service." Both of these are inherently "react and respond" oriented. When you study the best experience stagers, throughout all industries you see that they are clearly "anticipate and orchestrate" oriented. Yet only 30% of respondents defined patient experience as an aligned set of activities in support of a meaningfully customized experience.

The story in the stone: Patient experience is a high priority weighed down by old concepts.

Measurement stuck in the past

Finally, the majority of respondents reported that their organization measures the success or failure of patient experience initiatives through existing patient satisfaction survey instruments. Although this practice is understandable, it is also confining and provides measurement from a single lens. It ties patient experience more strongly to its past than to its future. How do you measure anticipation, orchestration, and customization with current react-and-respond instruments? How do you gauge the whole of the experience, including the time and space before the patient arrives and after he or she departs the facility? And how do you measure whether meaning was dispensed with the medicine? If we are ever to think of it differently, we must measure it differently.

The story in the stone: New experience expectations will require new experience actions. New experience actions will require new experience measures.

The Journey from Aspiring to Accomplished

Unless they are addressed, the highs and lows reported in the survey will prevent patient experience from moving out of the early stages of an aspiring society and into the latter stages of an accomplished one.

Perhaps by studying the approach to quality in 1969 we can learn some things that will inform the approach to patient experience in 2009. No one in healthcare would have said 40 years ago that quality was anything other than a top priority, yet the practices, systems, budget, and managerial focus were nowhere near what they are now. Patient experience today finds itself in much the same place. Ironically, healthcare leaders are increasingly realizing that true quality is more than clinical outcomes—it cannot exist without experience quality. So until we invest the money and mental capital to make patient experience intentionally orchestrated, personally customized, relationship oriented, facility and technology anticipated, storytelling inspired, and constantly taught and lived by leaders, healthcare won't progress beyond its current point on the learning curve.

Many lessons beyond those mentioned here are contained in the rock of this groundbreaking dig. But although the study answers a lot of the questions about the patient experience circa 2010, it poses some, too. In 2050, will we still be an aspiring society seeking to find a method to make our patient experience aspirations real? Will we have slipped backward into survival mode, succumbing to the lurking dangers of a broken system? Or will 2010 be that stratification in the rock that will show healthcare "archaeologists" of the future exactly when healthcare

leaders refused to keep playing it safe, devoted themselves to staging an intentionally meaningful patient experience, and invested their talents and treasures to
build an accomplished society that changed the world? It can go forward from
here; it can go backward from here. So what will your patient experience legacy
be? What story will the stone of your organization tell?

IMMERSE YOURSELF:
The Best Way to Learn about Experiences

What is the best way to learn something new? The honest answer is that it depends on the subject. If it's multiplication, flash card memorization is the best method. If it's surgery, the "see one, do one, teach one" school has a lot to recommend it. But when it comes to the new world of business experiences, there is no better way than immersion (which is why we created the extensive CD-ROM materials for this book). The idea that experiences must be experienced to be understood may not sound particularly insightful at first. But because the hallmark of a great experience is an emotionally meaningful memory, logical and mental analytics, by itself, is not enough. A great example of the power of an immersive, intentionally orchestrated personal experience is the Holocaust Museum in Washington, DC. You can read about the Holocaust all you want. You could speak to the dwindling number of people who survived it. But there is nothing quite like the experience of going to the museum, being assigned an actual prisoner number, and journeying through the exhibit before finding out whether you (representing the prisoner whose number you were given) made it out alive. It changes your point of view forever.

Experience Expeditions

When we first work with people to help them transform themselves, their departments, and even their companies into successful experience stagers, we often take them on an "experience expedition." These journeys take place in their own hometown or in an experience hub such as New York City; Orlando, FL; or Chicago. The purpose of the expeditions is to expose people, firsthand, to businesses that have achieved a substantial differentiation through their concentration on experience design and staging. We combine guided, drop-in visits with some in-depth backstage interviews with company executives. Participants extract best principles, not best practices, to apply in their truly groundbreaking work. We mix up the businesses we study, but we do go to the smash Broadway hit *Wicked* whenever possible. What is it about that particular show that is so important that we always include it in our expeditions, even though it often means paying triple the face value for tickets? Well, if you've seen the show, you know its production values, choreography, and music are out of this world. It teaches the important principle of onstage and offstage performance. But we could get that in almost any Broadway production. What sets *Wicked* apart is the nature of its story and the lesson it has for all would-be experience stagers, especially those in healthcare: The play portrays in an unforgettable way how things change when you truly understand the life story of someone you are trying to serve, be it patient, family member, employee, physician, board member, donor, or volunteer. It can completely change your point of view about what's good and what's bad, what's acceptable and what's not.

 The Complete Guide to Transforming the Patient Experience

A Necessary Change

For a long time, healthcare has desperately needed a dramatic change in its point of view, if we are to believe the research conducted by healthcare marketers over the past 25 years. (And after 25 years of the same results, shouldn't we be well beyond questioning them by now?)

Healthcare, the most personal of all service businesses, is constantly described as impersonal and dehumanizing. In studies of local hospitals and regional health systems, national integrated providers, for-profit organizations, and nonprofit organizations, the results are always the same: impersonal; dehumanizing. Now, about the same time that this data was emerging, our baby boomer customers were telling us this perspective-changing story in a different and more powerful way than through focus groups and telephone surveys. Think back to the early 1980s. If we had really understood what was going on then, the transformation that healthcare needs would be much further along today. That's when baby boomers touched healthcare for the first time in significant numbers—when they started having babies of their own. And they expressed their expectations for what healthcare should be like in dramatic fashion. A physician-directed clinical service, performed with mom knocked out in the delivery room and dad handing out cigars in the waiting room, was no longer acceptable. Instead, they expected high-quality, clinically safe care. It was no more than table stakes. They expected, for the very first time in healthcare anywhere, a masterfully orchestrated, person-ally meaningful, highly customized, patient- and family-directed experience in a healing environment.

The baby boomer generation taught us almost 30 years ago what we are still learning today: The experience economy will require the transformation of healthcare, not the incremental improvement of healthcare. (Can you imagine, by the way, if you decided to blow off the experience demands of the baby boomers as extraneous fluff and continued delivering babies the same old way, thinking that only improving quality scores and patient outcomes data would provide the differentiation your hospital would need to be successful? What outcomes data are there for a service line with 0% market share?)

Unfortunately, we didn't understand the lessons the baby boomers were imparting about their healthcare, so although we changed obstetrics, we kept everything else the same. After all, OB was just the "happy" service; it wasn't really serious medicine, such as cardiology, surgery, and oncology.

Again and again, starting in the late 1970s, baby boomers have tried to educate healthcare about fitness centers, spas, health food, cosmetic surgery, dietary supplements, acupuncture, cosmetic dentistry, veterinary medicine, and a whole variety of health-related services. But mostly we missed the lessons and, unfortunately, the revenue.

Recently, they gave us one more chance to get it right, this time on behalf of their parents, by introducing us to concepts such as hospice care. Think about the qualities of a hospice: It is a masterfully orchestrated, personally meaningful, highly customized, patient- and family-directed experience in a healing environment. It is not an impersonal, dehumanizing disassembly of institutions and professionals that too often require the constant monitoring by a patient advocate because, left to its own devices, it seems to conspire against the best interests of the patient. Whenever we get dismayed that healthcare will stay at the bottom of the experience class with other remedial learners such as the airlines and car companies, we are comforted by this one important statistic: Every 11 seconds another baby boomer turns 60. Now on the verge of their prime healthcare-consuming years, there is no doubt that healthcare will be transformed into an experience, whether healthcare leaders want to help or not.

For those leaders who do want to help and who see that their legacy and their institution's survival depend on it, understanding the nature of experiences and the requirements for successfully staging them has become the most important learning of their entire careers. As you can tell from the foreword to this book, we are big fans of Joe Pine and Jim Gilmore. Their book *The Experience Economy* is required reading for anyone in healthcare who wants to lead the experience revolution. They define experience from the customer's point of view. "Experiences are inherently personal, existing only in the mind of an individual who has been engaged on an emotional, physical, intellectual, or even spiritual level," they write. From an economic point of view, they define a staged experience as "a distinct class of economic offering that is as distinct from delivered services as delivered services are from the manufactured goods and the agricultural commodities that preceded them." This insight is crucial because it means that experiences are not the latest and greatest improvement in customer service; they are something altogether different.

Experiences Are Everywhere

Although goods are made and services are delivered, experiences are staged. This will require fundamentally new methods to be used, methods more akin to those taught in the theater department than in the business school.

FROM COMMODITY TO TRANSFORMATION

For the first of what will be many times during your reading of this book, we ask you to go to the Learning Curve CD-ROM included with this book. Open the "Chapter 2" folder and click on "CAKE" to watch Joe Pine take you through the progression of the economic value of a birthday cake from commodity to good to service to experience and, finally, to transformation. You'll use this great example many times to explain your new work of experience design and staging to others.

Go ahead. We'll wait.

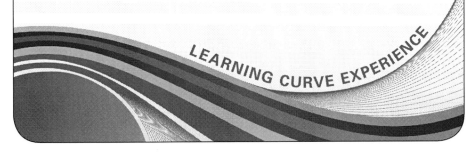

Now that you understand more clearly that the rise of customized, staged experiences is not only a way to avoid commoditization but also a way to differentiate yourself in the marketplace and enjoy premium pricing for your offerings, you are probably more interested in studying its applications in a wide variety of businesses. And there are numerous examples in just about every size and type of business that exists.

 The Complete Guide to Transforming the Patient Experience

ARE YOU EXPERIENCED?

Not quite convinced that experiences are everywhere and not the sole domain of entertainment and retail?

Do you remember that experience expedition we referenced at the beginning of this chapter? Well, you may not have realized that you've been conducting your own, albeit unguided and unintentional, version of one ever since the turn of the century. Want proof? Go again to the Learning Curve CD-ROM included with this book. Open the "Chapter 2" folder and click on "QUIZ" to take the "Are You Experienced?" quiz. Make sure to follow the instructions carefully.

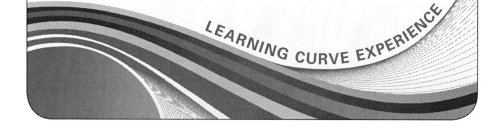

LEARNING CURVE EXPERIENCE

What did you notice from doing this exercise? What lessons can we learn from the businesses in the quiz? For starters, experiences come in all shapes, sizes, and price points. They are in every industry, even business-to-business. (We could have included hundreds more examples, but we thought 64 made the point.) These companies are dramatically different. Their customers describe them with enthusiasm. They also make customers want to spend more time there. After all, going beyond just a quick in-and-out transaction was one of the secrets to Starbucks' early success, wasn't it?

Had you done this exercise in a group, you would have also noticed that whether you checked the greatest number of experiences or the least, you would be an enthusiastic teacher of the lessons exemplified in your favorite experience. Finally, you would have observed that some people loved experiences you didn't think were that great or maybe that you even disliked—proving the point that experiences are personal.

By immersing yourself in these experience businesses, whether through expedition or exercise, you will have more fully grasped the lessons of our favorite Broadway musical and have begun laying the foundation for a lasting competitive advantage for your organization that is truly *Wicked*.

The Rise of the Talent Agency

The experience economy will not only change what companies do on the outside for customers, it will also change the very way traditional management functions are performed inside those companies. Let's look at how the collision with the experience economy will fundamentally change one traditional management function: human resources (HR).

If experiences are staged (and they are), and if authentically staging them will require a thoughtful and intentional employee experience (which it will), then HR departments of the future will function more like talent agencies and less like policy police. They will carefully audition prospective employees, looking well beyond specific job-related training and experience to their ability to perform in a particular role as directed by the intentional theme of the business. The motivation of their role and its choreography with other roles will be clearly explained in something that looks and feels much different from anything that is contained in present-day new employee orientation.

In the future, department directors and supervisors will continuously rehearse their employees' performance. Training and development will go beyond the occasional program sponsored by the education department. A new role, that of "talent agent," will be common in HR departments. Every morning, they'll wake up thinking about how they can help their specific portfolio of "employee clients" to develop into more valuable, more skilled, and more enthusiastically committed performers. Evaluations, awards, education, and benefits will be customized to each individual. Each employee's assignments will be designed to spur his or her growth. As you can see, this is not an HR department that is slightly friendlier and just a little more responsive. It is fundamentally different—all because of the fundamentally different requirements of the experience economy. This kind of change will be felt throughout healthcare in strategy, finance, IT, facilities design, marketing, and every patient contact and ancillary support department.

The Sharp Experience

Staging experiences is not just another management thing to do; it is a new way of doing all management. It transforms managers into leaders.

Sharp HealthCare is a prime example of how an organizationwide focus on experience transforms all aspects of a healthcare system—from employee engagement and education to customer interaction and marketing. Sharp is a nonprofit, fully integrated healthcare system in San Diego, operating seven hospitals and two affiliated medical groups and offering a full array of healthcare programs and services. Sharp has more than 30 different physical locations and counts among its associates 14,000 team members, 2,600 affiliated physicians, and 2,000 volunteers. As such, Sharp is San Diego's largest health system and largest private employer.

As with many other healthcare systems, the early 1990s brought Sharp HealthCare significant growth, along with financial and operational challenges. In the mid-1990s, the board and leadership team refocused the organization from its growth strategy to an operations strategy. This required many difficult changes, including selling and closing certain operations and implementing a very rigorous financial discipline. By 2000, Sharp enjoyed a financially healthy bottom line and a rating as the number one health system in California (Modern Healthcare, February/March 2000). It was then that Sharp made a significant commitment to and investment in experiences.

Although it would have been easy to consider the turnaround and national accolades a signal that Sharp was in great shape, instead the organization took its success as the impetus to listen to the voice of the customer. Sharp took a cue from Jim Collins and his book *Good to Great* to determine what Sharp could do to move from being a good organization to a great one.

Sharp focus

In late 2000, Sharp commissioned 100 focus groups of key stakeholders, including employees, physicians, and patient groups. Even with all of the research available, there's nothing quite as valuable as the direct feedback from your employees, physicians, and customers to light a fire for change. The purpose of these focus groups was to gain insight into the overall experience at Sharp from the point of view of team members, physician partners, and patients. The feedback was clear and consistent. Each constituent group shared that the experience at Sharp was "just okay." It was really no different from any other healthcare experience—clinically sound and efficient, but lacking in warmth, anticipation, or personalization. They were clear that there was much room for improvement. Not only did these focus groups reveal an opportunity for experience improvement at Sharp, but participants also shared that healthcare as an industry had much room for improvement, too.

Sharp faced a difficult dilemma: hold on to the industry accolades and ignore the direct feedback from key constituents (what some might have considered the easy way out), or take the feedback as a gift and use it as a catalyst for organizational (and, hopefully, industrywide) transformation. The Sharp leadership team made a huge commitment to invest time and resources to improve the organization by improving the experience for employees, physicians, and patients. This meant getting better at every level, from employee interaction and engagement to process improvement and purposeful experience design.

The concept of experiences and the experience economy was quite new at this time, so a small, multidisciplinary team of Sharp leaders (from frontline managers to hospital administrators and the system CEO) set out on a best practice investigation to determine what the best of the best—across all industries—were doing to create truly memorable employee and customer experiences. The first stop on the six-month investigation was Pine and Gilmore's thinkAbout—a two-day immersive learning event designed to impart the principles of the experience economy (where, by the way, Gary and Sonia first met). The Sharp team also learned from Disney, Ritz-Carlton, General Electric, and the Studer Group.

Sharp vision

Ultimately, the investigation sparked an organizationwide performance improvement initiative called The Sharp Experience—complete with a new organizational vision and a new model for change.

Sharp's vision was to transform the healthcare experience and make Sharp the best place to work, the best place to practice medicine, and the best place to receive care. Ultimately, Sharp set its sights on creating the best healthcare system in the universe.

The model for The Sharp Experience consists of three core components:

- Experience and performance improvement, designed to actively engage team members, at all levels, in creating positive change related to the workplace experience and the customer experience

- Accountability systems and structures, ensuring alignment of goals across the organization, along with systems and structures of accountability

- Learning and development, which launched The Sharp University, a corporate university designed to provide education and development for leaders, team members, and affiliated physicians

Fundamental to the initiative were the discovery and belief that focusing first on the employee experience and the overall culture would enable comprehensive customer experience improvement and overall organizational outcomes. Sharp's transformation required thinking anew about all aspects of the organization, and the work to intentionally create the best healthcare experiences, happened outside the traditional departments and structures. Originally born out of the marketing division, Sharp soon developed a new internal competency focused specifically on employee engagement, culture change, and experience design. Once begun, the momentum was unstoppable—the difference was palpable. Employees and customers alike began to tell stories of The Sharp Experience. And those stories ultimately became the basis for a one-of-a-kind reality-based marketing strategy that garnered unprecedented results.

Sharp results

An intentional, purpose-filled focus on the employee experience and the customer experience drives more than just positive feelings. As a result of The Sharp Experience, Sharp HealthCare has improved year over year on every single measure and metric—from quality outcomes, market share, and patient satisfaction to net revenue, turnover, and employee satisfaction. Although there will always be work to do to create employee and customer experiences that surpass ever-escalating expectations, Sharp's progress to date earned the organization the 2007 Malcolm Baldrige National Quality Award, the nation's highest presidential honor for organizational excellence. Now that's an experience!

AN EXPERIENCE MARRIAGE:
Marketing and Operations Together at Last

A change in point of view as big as what we've described will take a fundamental redefinition of just about everything, including new leadership roles, new management skills, and new personal commitments. This is transformational work, not incremental improvement work, and nowhere will the changes be felt more profoundly than in the marketing development of a healthcare company. Why is that? There are two reasons. First, because marketing is still a relatively new management discipline in healthcare (the first marketing titles and departments started showing up in hospitals in the early 1980s), it has been a sporadically budgeted, mostly reactionary function that has too often been driven more by politics than by brand strategy. Although there are obvious and brilliant exceptions to this assessment, if you step back and objectively analyze the entire body of work produced over the past 25 years, we think you'll come to a conclusion that is, if not in total agreement, at least in the same ZIP code as ours.

Historically, and across the majority of healthcare organizations, marketing expenditures are typically at the top on the chopping block when times get tough financially. You could blame the fact that most health administration curricula—even today's—don't contain much meaningful study of marketing, and therefore healthcare leaders don't understand it nearly as well as finance, management, human resources, strategy, or facilities design. Or you could blame healthcare marketing professionals for too often staying in their communications comfort zone and thereby abdicating their vital strategic connection to operations. You could also blame physicians who expect that marketing support of their service lines and their egos be doled out as candy rewards to the health system's most favored children. There are many causes for healthcare marketing's history of underperformance and many who could share in the blame.

But the point here is not to place blame; it is to acknowledge what is and to acknowledge that marketing, as it is widely practiced in healthcare today, will not succeed in the experience economy.

And that brings us to our second reason for the belief that profound changes are coming to marketing and branding in healthcare: Experiences are staged.

Think about the implications of those three words for just a minute. They mean there must be consistent intention. There has to be flawless orchestration. And most importantly, this intention and orchestration must live in operations, not just communications. Gone are the days when the brand promise can be a whole lot better than the brand experience. (You know from personal experience that if you could check into the ads of most hospitals, it would be a lot better than checking into the actual hospital itself.) Gone too are the days when healthcare marketing professionals can concern themselves primarily with well-designed campaigns instead of well-designed experiences.

So how do we make the shift that will be required to succeed? Well, it makes sense that if your brand will have to live in both the world of communications and the world of operations, the changes will have to be evident in both words and actions. Let's start with words.

The Power of Words

One good thing about the rise of the experience economy over the past 10 years is that the word *experience* is a lot more prevalent in business now than it was back then. To say you were in experience design and staging in 2000 was to instantly elicit quizzical looks and pointed questions about when you were going to get a real job. But now all that has changed. There was the bestselling success of the book *The Experience Economy* in 1999. *Fast Company* magazine designated "experience designer" as its Number 1 hot job in 2007. And *Time* magazine labeled authentic experience design and staging as one of its "Ten Ideas That Are Changing the World" in 2008.

But as in most things, exploding popularity has its dark side, and the dark side here is that it's a lot easier to say the word *experience* than do the work of experience. So you see customer service become customer experience in the blink of an eye. Customer relationship management departments become customer experience management departments literally overnight. And yet none of the function actually changes; it just sounds like the work got a whole lot cooler and hipper. It won't be long before it becomes evident that we've changed the wrapper but not what's inside. And when the results that healthcare leaders hoped for fail to materialize, everyone will get impatient when the latest magic bullet fails to make them rich or famous.

As a healthcare professional who is deeply interested and invested in the success of the healthcare industry, you know better than most the power of words to direct and inspire action. That's what the saying "The pen is mightier than the sword" means. In addition to the cautions noted earlier, there is one more when it comes to experiential or experience-based marketing. That's it. Right there. Did you see it? It's using some form of the word *experience* as an adjective to modify the word *marketing*. This may seem like a trivial thing, until you consider the answer to this question: Does implementing experiential marketing differ from creating marketing experiences? You bet it does, because experiential marketing is only one of a number of different types of marketing you could employ. There's target marketing, niche marketing, direct marketing, outdoor marketing, in-home marketing, Internet marketing, strategic marketing, relationship marketing, media marketing, guerilla marketing, partner marketing, and cause-related marketing, to name a few. The problem with these words is that they immediately turn experience into something tactical. It's just another thing to do instead of a new way of doing all things. In healthcare, this problem is multiplied because of the unfortunate view that marketing is synonymous with communications, so experiential marketing becomes just another way to get the word out, albeit in a more interactive way.

In 2002, Joe Pine and Jim Gilmore put forth the phrase "the experience IS the marketing" in a whitepaper by the same name. Its advice to all businesses is that "the best way to market any offering (good, service, or experience) is with an experience so engaging that potential customers can't help but pay attention— and pay up as a result ... people have become relatively immune to messages targeted at them. The best way to reach your customers is to create an experience within them."

To underscore the distinction between experience marketing and marketing experiences, Pine and Gilmore proposed one simple guideline that put a new spin on an old Peter Drucker saying: "The aim of experiences is to make marketing superfluous."

The Bridge from Words to Action

Marketing experiences are the way to make healthcare marketing operational in its focus and intentional in its purpose. They are the bridge from words to actions. And they are the multiplying reinforcement of all the communications work your organization does. (Remember, the number of people someone tells about a bad experience is far greater than the number of people someone tells about a good one.) This is why the airlines and healthcare continue in a downward spiral. There are just too many bad experiences for any advertising to credibly overcome. Let's take a look at this insight in action.

In the late 1990s, Sharp HealthCare followed the traditional route to marketing the organization—a combination of brand and call-to-action advertising, communications, and interactive customer touch points, including a call center and comprehensive Web site. Advertising strategy and execution were relatively traditional, with high production–value television and radio ads and a complementary print strategy. Although very attractive to look at, the reality was that these glossy ads did not effectively differentiate the organization from the competition. In marketing efforts throughout the region and across the nation, healthcare organizations were telling consumers that they were "the biggest," "the first," "the most," and "the best." In actuality, the majority of healthcare advertising campaigns were so similar that the organizations' names could have been interchangeable—and research showed that in the minds of consumers, that was often the case.

The growth of the Internet in the late 1990s provided a new platform for marketing—a new method for differentiation—and at Sharp, it wasn't long before the company created a comprehensive consumer Web site that presented new insight into the interactive, individual healthcare experience that customers sought. The Web allowed the organization to anticipate needs, personalize information, and communicate and engage in meaningful, immediate dialogues. How ironic that an industry built on human, face-to-face, personal interactions was finding greater depth and connectivity through the Web. These online chats and e-mails pulled back the curtain on the difference between the experience that customers were seeking at a hospital or healthcare provider and the experience they were actually having when at a hospital or healthcare provider. So the Internet created a grand new venue for providing deep, rich healthcare information and interaction at the same time that it magnified the chasm that was growing between customer desire and customer experience.

The Internet was offering opportunities for improvement, but the key in-person healthcare experiences were still more likely to be exasperating than not. They were still composed of processes designed for the healthcare system rather than patients and families. The reality was that healthcare was confusing, complex, and cumbersome. Friends, neighbors, and team members alike began to share frustrations, ask for guidance and assistance, or just break down about their experiences. These frustrations were mostly not about clinical expertise or outcomes—rather, they were about how a healthcare experience made them feel as human beings.

The Internet served as a new conduit for better understanding our customers and sparking organizational change, and it also served as a sober reminder that an organization's story and message no longer remained in the control of a marketing department. With the click of a mouse, each individual's healthcare experience could be told to thousands or even millions of people, with the ability to squash any advertising or public relations campaign.

This confluence of factors, along with the results of the stakeholder focus groups, compelled the marketing leaders at Sharp to learn everything they could about staging and creating meaningful experiences.

When your staff, physicians, and patients are all telling you that the experience is "just okay"—and really no different from any other healthcare organization—it's a call to action. A call to action that made it virtually impossible to continue the tried-and-true marketing campaigns when there was such a disconnect between the story we told about the organization and the experience customers had with the organization (and the resulting story they told about us).

Some organizations might simply take this information and use it to inform a newly crafted ad campaign. They mistakenly think that if patients want a better healthcare experience, the solution is to create a campaign that tells people their experience is the best without actually doing the work to make the experience the best. But the leaders at Sharp took a different stand. They knew they could not continue marketing the organization unless the organization had a very different story to tell. The new story needed to start from within—from the experience that was created and staged each and every day with each and every patient or customer interaction. The Sharp team understood that true marketing starts at the bedside (in Pine and Gilmore's terms, "the experience IS the marketing"). And the authenticity and credibility of the story and any marketing campaign required complete alignment between brand promise and brand experience.

To ensure that all of Sharp's leaders understood the significance of the feedback and the gap between customer desire and customer experience, Sharp's marketing leaders took a bold step and suggested that the annual budget for advertising be allocated to improving the healthcare experience. They knew an investment in the experience would allow for far greater differentiation in any future marketing efforts. What a concept!

Here's the lesson we can learn from Sharp and other healthcare organizations that are getting experience right: Let's not continue to tell the same old story. Let's transform every aspect of the healthcare experience so that we can tell a new story—a story that will resonate with patients and caregivers alike. A story that could spark customers to tell our story for us.

Sharp's leaders blurred the lines between operations and marketing as they orchestrated and led an organizationwide performance through an experience improvement initiative that came to be known as The Sharp Experience. After studying the best of the best in employee and customer experience design, the team developed a model to transform the healthcare experience at Sharp.

EXPERIENCE DRIVERS:
From the Inside Out and the Outside In

Creating an altogether different (and better) healthcare experience for patients and customers does more than improve customer satisfaction scores. A focus on experience improvement has the ability to make the entire organization better. That's because transforming the healthcare experience for patients and customers is greatly aided by a focus and commitment to transforming the healthcare experience for employees and physicians—the caregivers. By focusing on creating the very best caregiver experience, a new-to-the-world patient experience can emerge and be more reliably sustainable. It's an inside-out improvement process.

Companies and leaders often say, "Our people are our greatest asset." Unfortunately, the claim is often more talk than action—more fiction than reality. People know whether you value them by how you treat them—by the experience you create for them and with them—not because you simply tell them they are the company's "greatest asset." The rhetoric fools no one.

Successful businesses and brands know that bottom-line results aren't possible without wholehearted employee engagement. The *Gallup Management Journal* publishes a semiannual Employee Engagement Index and the most recent U.S. results indicate the following:

- 29% of employees are actively engaged in their jobs. These employees work with passion and feel a profound connection to their company. People who are actively engaged help move the organization forward.

- 54% of employees are not engaged. These employees have essentially "checked out" or "retired in place," moving through the paces, putting the time but not the passion into their work.

- 17% of employees are actively disengaged. These employees are like a cancer in the organization, undermining the accomplishments of engaged coworkers and acting out their unhappiness.

These figures should be a wake-up call to all leaders and organizations. The experience economy calls for businesses to create positively memorable experiences and engage customers in an inherently personal way. As such, the role of the employee evolves from service provider to experience stager or personal guide. And to thrive in the experience economy, experiences must be rendered authentic—so the role of the employee as performer or guide is all the more critical.

Just as patients and customers are seeking personal, customized healthcare experiences, so too are employees seeking personal, customized employee experiences. It is virtually impossible to achieve breakthrough patient and customer experiences without a commitment to intentionally create and cultivate employee experiences.

Let's be clear. The employee experience is not the proverbial set of benefits offered by a company—healthcare and dental, 401k, incremental salary hikes—or even the elements touted in quarterly and annual reports. These are simply the "price of admission" in today's world. The employee experience that matters drives passion, purpose, and sense of ownership and engagement not through "stuff," but rather through vision, leadership, clarity, communication, and providing employees with a sense that their job has meaning and makes a difference.

The relationship between profit, employee engagement, and customer satisfaction was described very clearly in the classic business article, "The Service-Profit Chain," which was first published in the *Harvard Business Review* in 1994, stating:

> *Profit and growth are stimulated primarily by customer loyalty. Loyalty is a direct result of customer satisfaction. Satisfaction is largely influenced by the value of services provided to customers. Value is created by satisfied, loyal, and productive employees.*

If we were to update this description to create a more current experience-based version, it might look something like this (see Figure 4.1):

> *Profit and growth are stimulated by customer loyalty. Loyalty is a direct result of a positively memorable customer experience. The customer experience is largely influenced by the value of the experience staged—for customers by employees. Value is created by passionate, purpose-filled, engaged employees.*

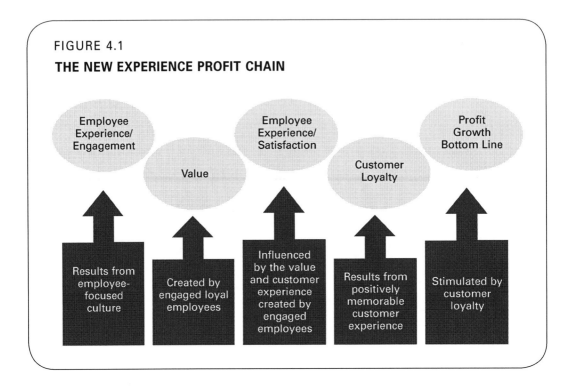

FIGURE 4.1

THE NEW EXPERIENCE PROFIT CHAIN

Walt Disney captured this concept very simply in a quote often attributed to him:

You can design and create and build the most wonderful place in the world. But it takes people to make the dream a reality.

When companies intentionally design and cultivate a personal, meaningful employee experience, they will be rewarded with a workforce that is no longer just active but aligned; no longer just compliant but committed; no longer just productive but passionate.

Understanding that organizational success (the bottom line) is driven by engaged employees (the frontline) is core to understanding the power and importance of a deliberate employee experience. The competence and skills of employees; their enthusiasm, motivation, and loyalty; the spirit with which they interact among themselves and with patients and customers; their willingness to support and work by organizational vision and standards; the empowerment they get from their leaders; the overall culture—are all crucial to an exceptional customer experience driving productivity, innovation, and growth.

Engaging Employees at Sharp HealthCare

For Sharp HealthCare, their nationwide best practice investigation sparked the discovery and belief that focusing first on the employee experience and the overall culture would drive the customer experience and overall organizational outcomes with the aim of achieving the vision of transforming the healthcare experience and making Sharp the best place to work, practice medicine, and receive care.

It's one thing to create a new vision, new structure, and new model for change, but with 14,000 employees in more than 30 locations, the key would be to engage the entire workforce in the transformation. Sharp team members would be the key, and The Sharp Experience was designed to focus first on creating the best environment and experience for employees so that they could together create the best experience for patients.

The Sharp Experience was launched in 2001 with a one-of-a-kind event called the All-Staff Assembly. Every Sharp team member was transported by bus, train, or trolley to the San Diego Convention Center to hear President and CEO Mike Murphy share his new vision to transform the healthcare experience. The sessions were designed as recommitment assemblies—a time for the organization to come together to recommit to the purpose in their work and the difference they make in the lives of others—and to join together in creating a truly new healthcare experience.

The first All-Staff Assembly was so invigorating and inspiring that it has become an annual ritual, providing team members with time for inspiration, education, and celebration. Each event has a theme and is designed to encourage team members to share their spark of possibility with others. There's even a Sharp choir, made up of caregivers, physicians, and staff members, that sings its way into the souls of Sharp attendees.

'The Wisdom Is in This Room'

Embarking on a transformational journey is no small task, and getting team members on board would be critical to the success of the endeavor. At the first All-Staff Assembly sessions in 2001, team members learned of Sharp's new vision for the future. They were then asked to become the architects of change and create the experiences that would transform the organization and help make the vision a reality. The most powerful moment was when Murphy stood before the group and said, "We don't have all the answers or know exactly what it's going to take, and

I am going to need each of you to help. What I do know is that I'm confident that the wisdom is in this room—that the people of Sharp have the creativity, initiative, and expertise to make this happen."

It was with that call to action and clear statement of confidence that Sharp leaders and team members stepped forward. Overnight, more than 1,000 team members were actively engaged in formal "Action Teams" for change, focused on creating a great place for people to work and a great place for patients to receive care. Employee-based Action Teams created the core fundamentals of The Sharp Experience, including 12 standards of behavior that each and every employee is held accountable to, regardless of title or position.

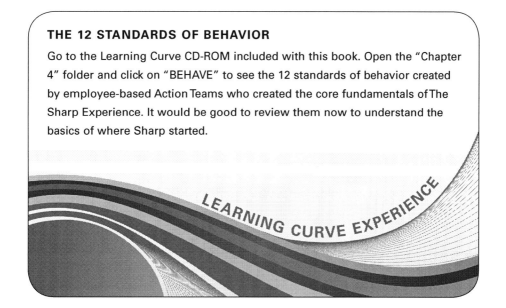

THE 12 STANDARDS OF BEHAVIOR

Go to the Learning Curve CD-ROM included with this book. Open the "Chapter 4" folder and click on "BEHAVE" to see the 12 standards of behavior created by employee-based Action Teams who created the core fundamentals of The Sharp Experience. It would be good to review them now to understand the basics of where Sharp started.

At its core, The Sharp Experience is about nurturing and crafting the culture of the organization. Engaging and exciting employees in a new vision and enlisting them to become architects of change has created an unstoppable momentum. The passion for creating the best employee experience fuels the passion for creating a truly transformative customer experience. Sharp team members frequently share that through The Sharp Experience they've become "better parents" and "better people," with a passion to make Sharp and the world a better place. What could be better than that?

A Fully Customized Experience

As if it wasn't enough that you had to study a whole new set of companies and master a whole new set of skills to create a new patient experience, now we're telling you that you have to create an intentional experience for each employee, too.

Do you have the feeling that your job of being a healthcare leader just got a whole lot bigger and more complex? It has. Are you concerned that you don't know how to do a lot of this new stuff? You should be. Are you tempted to just wait it out, thinking that healthcare is different or that your organization is different? Are you trying to convince yourself right now that your employees are "engaged enough" already? Are you hoping that the experience economy won't really apply to you? If so, you are heading in a dangerous direction. And here's why.

Experiences are not just being driven from the inside by increasing employee expectations. They are also being driven by some huge outside forces. We already showed you how the baby boomers have changed everything they've touched in and around healthcare into experiences, including obstetrics, fitness centers, spas, health food stores, hospices, and more. Do you think that will suddenly change now that they are on the verge of their prime healthcare consuming years? (We don't think so, either.)

We've also shown how experiences are transforming all other industries, not just entertainment and retail. There's Pike Place Fish Market in commodities, American Girl in manufactured goods, and Geek Squad in delivered services. There's Johnson Controls, TST Engineering, H+L Architecture, and Starizon in business-to-business experiences. There's Planet Ford in car repair, Crème de la Crème in daycare, the Library Hotel in hospitality, the Charmin Experience in toilet paper, Gumball Wizard in gumballs, Cerritos Library in nonprofits, Steinway in piano delivery, Whole Foods in grocery stores, and Apple in technology stores.

We could easily go on for several pages just listing all the things that have changed, and you still might not be convinced because this little voice in your head is saying that although those are great examples for other industries, they're not for healthcare because healthcare is different. For starters, no one wants to come to a hospital.

We could make the case that a number of the fish markets, computer repair services, grocery stores, engineering firms, consultants, and gumball and toilet paper manu-facturers don't have people clamoring to spend time with them either, but we won't. Instead, we'll offer up another example that by any measure is one that people don't want to be in: a car accident. If you look at what Progressive Casualty Insurance Company has done with its rapid response vehicles to transform what's brought to the site of an accident (everything including a cup of coffee, a cell phone, a tow truck, a rental car, an uplinked computerized claim estimation system, and even a check for the damages), it's clear that the experience economy has ventured far beyond the grounds at Disney. People are getting experiences everywhere and they will expect them in healthcare, too. So, now we have two pretty compelling reasons, but let's keep going.

Technology is another powerful trend fueling the proliferation of experiences, specifically something called Moore's Law, which states that every 20 years the cost of processing a single bit of information decreases by a factor of 1,000. But what does that have to do with experiences?

Remember how we said experiences are inherently personal and they have to engage you in a way that is meaningful and memorable? Moore's Law means that for the first time in human history, it is not too costly to remember important things about individual customers. As leaders, that means we no longer have to communicate at the level of the mass market or a segment or even a niche. We can meaningfully communicate at the level of the individual, and that changes everything (this is true on the employee level, too, even if you have 14,000 of them).

We can do much more than communicate in an individually meaningful way. We can also make products, deliver services, and stage experiences for customers in an individually meaningful way. That's why we've seen the explosion of customized experiences onto the scene in such a brief time. And if there is a lot of it now, consider how much more of it there will be in 20 years, when remembering things about individuals is

1,000 times cheaper than it is today. Even those of us who aren't very good at math know that it's a really big number.

Are you there yet? Fully committed to the fact that your life and career are about to change in a fabulous way? That creating patient and employee experiences will provide a new passion for your work as a leader? If not, don't worry, we've saved the best for last. It's more influential than the baby boomers and their love of experiences reaching their prime healthcare consuming years. It's more convincing than the transformation of an entire economy and every industry in it into predominantly experience-based offerings. It's more powerful than the implication of the mathematical magic of Moore's Law. It is the most personal technology ever invented, and it is being invented in healthcare as you read this. Further, it can't succeed without being surrounded by a personalized experience. What is it? It's gene-based medicine.

Personal Medicine in an Impersonal Way

Genetic medicine is based entirely on the idea that we can go beyond treating cancer, for example, to treating the cancer in you. Precisely. Exactly. Genetically. Can this most personal of all technologies, one that purports to know you and act on your behalf at the level of your chromosomes, be delivered effectively in the current impersonal and dehumanizing way? Not a chance. So unless we want to hold back the biggest breakthrough in the history of medicine, we better get busy creating an experience revolution worthy of the scientific one that is already underway. And to do this, we'll have to go way beyond the recent, well-intentioned interest in improving our hospital's relative rank in customer satisfaction.

Experience is not service on steroids

When the Hospital Consumer Assessment of Healthcare Providers and Systems, better known as HCAHPS, came out, there was an understandable surge in interest in improving customer service. After all, if the general public can now easily see how patients and families rate their experience, they might choose to go elsewhere. That's pretty motivating. Why did the data from this national standardized survey of patients' perceptions of their hospital experience become a motivator only when others could see it? What happened to the idea that your high school report card didn't have to be posted throughout the whole school for it to motivate you? And how did 60% come to be considered a "good" score anyway? These are obvious questions that come to mind as hospitals race to justify or improve their scores. What's also obvious is that improvement in customer service in healthcare is necessary, it's just not sufficient. A customized, personally meaningful, staged experience will beat a fast, friendly, generic delivered service 95% of the time. But it's not only that. It's where the service level currently is in healthcare that dooms a customer service improvement strategy almost from the start. We want you to think of an experience that has the following characteristics, which are typical to healthcare:

- You are stripped of your clothing and personal effects

- You are assigned a number

- You are made to wear embarrassing clothing

- You have spartan surroundings

- You are assigned a roommate you don't want

     The Complete Guide to Transforming the Patient Experience

- You have strict limitations on your visitors

- You have strict limitations on information

- You are admitted and discharged at the beginning and end of your stay

- You are served bland, institutional food

- Once you get out, you never want to go back

As you no doubt noticed, the healthcare experience sounds an awful lot like prison. And no amount of making a faster, better, cheaper version will ever be nearly enough.

So there you have it. Whether you start on the inside and work your way out or on the outside and work your way in, there can be no doubt that the experience economy is coming to healthcare. It's not a question of if; it's just a question of when.

STORIES MATTER:
How Leaders Can Convey Meaning and Drive Decisions

Stories matter. Stories in healthcare matter a lot—whether a person is telling the story of his or her healthcare experience as a patient or whether a healthcare organization is telling the story of its organization or brand. Through story, we bring meaning to our life experiences and fortify our memories. Stories, quite simply, are the way we remember things.

Think about the stories that people tell about healthcare today. Precious few stories regale positive details and enthusiastic endorsement. The vast majority of healthcare stories told today are negative. The media has a much greater appetite for the negative in healthcare. They love to report on bad outcomes, wrong-site surgery, medication mistakes, malpractice, and the ever-escalating price of care and treatment. These negative media stories captivate an audience and create a ripple effect. They incite people to share their own personal healthcare experiences, and even if the healthcare outcome was positive (successful surgery, healthy baby, heroics in the emergency department), personal healthcare stories tend to focus on dissatisfaction.

Stories about personal healthcare experiences stick in people's minds and hearts for a long time. They can often be summoned instantaneously and they transport people back in time to the very moment the experience took place. Ask people to tell a story about a healthcare experience and you are likely to get a raw, real narrative about far more than clinical procedures. Their cheeks may flush, their eyes may fill with tears, and they will undoubtedly share a gripping account of the emotions and feelings the experience triggered. Feelings such as embarrassment, frustration, anger, humiliation, or fear. They may start their stories with "You won't believe what happened to me." Or ask questions such as "Why do they make it so hard and confusing?" Or pronounce verdicts such as "It was a living nightmare."

Because stories have power, convey meaning, and can drive decision-making, it is critical for healthcare leaders to take a stand to creating a new story for healthcare. A new healthcare story starts from within an organization by engaging and exciting the healthcare workforce in intentionally crafting and creating truly personal and meaningful experiences for their patients and guests. Designing and staging positive healthcare experiences will begin to elicit more positive emotions surrounding the total healthcare experience—both for team members and for customers. These positive experiences and emotions will change the types of stories that team members will tell to patients and customers and the kind of story that patients and customers will tell to the world.

The Five Story Types

Storytelling will be the new healthcare marketing, thanks to the baby boom and the experience economy. But creating advertising, Web sites, and publications that include stories and testimonials is not enough. That's only a tiny part of what we have in mind. When we say storytelling is the new healthcare marketing, we are not talking about a semantic difference or a slight alteration of conventional practice. Rather, the storytelling we are talking about is much closer to that practiced by the first great experience stager in business, Walt Disney, when he opened his first theme park in 1955.

The real breakthrough Disney made then was to immerse his customers in a vibrant, engaging, and meaningful story. And just like the ones he had shown on TV and in theaters, every part either added to or subtracted from the story's power and its dramatic structure. How employees were hired was a story. How trash was picked up was a story. How buildings were designed and maintained was a story. How customers waited in line was a story. How and where the characters appeared was a story. What employees were called, how they were trained, and even how they got to their work stations was a story. How laundry was prepared was a story. What employees did for distressed or challenging guests was a story. The list goes on and on. Not only were each of these elements dynamic in their own right, but they were connected by a theme (hence the name *theme park*) in a way that was, shall we say, nothing short of "magical." Nothing was overlooked or unimportant. The attention to operational detail, purpose, and meaning was exquisite.

About the only thing that was regrettable, in Disney's eyes, were the intrusions on the story by the businesses that sprung up just outside Disneyland's gates that distracted mightily from the intended story immersions. So when he had the chance to do it again, he fixed that problem by buying 47 square miles in Florida and creating a "world" that is all its own.

You probably noticed that in the list of examples we used, we didn't mention Disney's advertising or promotion. Those are story laden, too, but that is much less unusual, much less remarkable. No, it's the operational stories, those told by actions, activities, props, and processes, that are the real key here. It is helping to construct these operational stories that will finally take healthcare marketing out of its diminished role as a communications-only support function. Even more important, it will take the healthcare industry out of its diminished role as a poorly run, not-to-be-emulated business sector.

There are five types of stories that successful healthcare leaders will help to conceive, write, perform, tell, and celebrate. We'll discuss each type in more detail in upcoming chapters. But for now, here is a brief summary:

- **Context stories:** a new and immersive way of developing and communicating the strategy of a healthcare organization

- **Personal stories:** a new and immersive way of creating culture by shining a vibrant and consistent light on the real stories of healthcare's everyday heroes

- **Powerful ceremonies:** a new and immersive way of creating, celebrating, and capturing meaning in the work of healthcare

- **Spatial stories:** a new and immersive way of designing and propping health-care buildings that transforms a mundane space into a memorable place for patients, families, physicians, and staff members

- **Rich traditions:** a new and immersive way of connecting all the other kinds of stories to create a powerful legacy that everyone feels lucky to be a part of

Imagination and Feeling

Maybe the most important word in that last sentence is *feels*, because healthcare has too often become unfeeling. Unfeeling to managers who bury themselves in the numbers. Unfeeling to patients who are treated as uninvolved subjects. Unfeeling to families who are treated as barely tolerated intrusions. Unfeeling to doctors who are disillusioned that all their training has led them to be well-paid assembly line workers. Unfeeling to nurses who are relegated to pass meds and fill out forms. Unfeeling to donors whose important contributions are monotonously recognized with another shovel, another ribbon cutting, another silent auction, or another name plaque. And unfeeling to talented students who increasingly see healthcare as one of the last places they would want to work. Impersonal, dehumanizing, and unfeeling for customers and workers—hardly the recipe for greatness. It is the ultimate irony; an industry dedicated to life is itself too often lifeless. It must stop.

That's why the future work of healthcare leaders is so vital. It's because great stories and great storytellers do two indispensable things that healthcare desperately needs: capture your imagination and make you feel. And because they unite the head and the heart, they can transform lifeless jobs into a life's work. Stories transform healthcare from the institutional to the inspirational. But to be believed, they must be operational, not just "orational." The old saying is true: "Most people would rather see a sermon than hear one any day." And whether your stories are told by your places, your people, or your policies, they must be told with the same passion and commitment on the hundredth time as they were the first time. Your stories, in all their forms, can be a living history of how a group of people decided to dispense sacredness with their surgery, dreams with their diagnostics, meaning with their medicine. Or it could be a living history of how a group of people saw a broken and dysfunctional healthcare system and decided to do nothing about it. And remember, no decision is a decision. So which will it be? Which way from your current point on the learning curve will you go? If it's the first, please read on. If it's the second, please stop complaining.

 The Complete Guide to Transforming the Patient Experience

A QUESTION OF GREATNESS:
Set a New Cultural Expectation

If healthcare leaders want their organizations to be truly great, what is the most important question they must consistently answer? We are not talking about being better than average. Our aspiration doesn't even stop at merely good. In fact, we agree with Jim Collins that "good is the enemy of great." Rather, we are talking about greatness that goes far beyond what was thought to be possible in healthcare: an organizational performance that sets new standards and a personal connection to the work that feels more like cause than career.

Asking the Right Question

When you think about it, most companies do a decent job of answering the "what" of their business. What industry are we in? What competition do we face? What customers do we serve? What do we extract, produce, deliver, stage, or guide? What do we expect financially? And so on. Answering such "what" questions, although important, can never by itself lead to greatness because the answers are merely descriptive, not distinctive.

So if "what" is not the question that leads to greatness, maybe we should be asking "how." This competency question starts to take us from the realm of the general to that of the specific. How do I perform this procedure? How do I enter the patient's room? How do I treat my colleagues? How do we evaluate performance? How do we develop and protect our brand?

Companies with the same answer to the question "what?" can have very different answers to the question "how?" Unique processes, approaches, and systems are all elements of how. Taken together, they describe the distinctive competence needed for a company to be good—maybe even very good. But not great. Why not? Thoreau had it right when he said, "Nothing great has ever been accomplished without enthusiasm." Asking "how?" does not generate any emotion, much less enthusiasm. It is necessary for greatness, it just isn't sufficient.

"Why?" is the question that generates understanding and commitment. It's a question that connects the heart with the head. "Why?" challenges conventional wisdom and inspires every breakthrough idea. "Why?" takes us beyond return on investment to return on involvement. It is the key to a vibrant culture, one that happily holds unreasonable expectations of itself and embraces change. Just imagine how different your recruitment, orientation, and training would be if you answered these "why" questions. Why do we look way beyond credentials and training in hiring the people who work here? Why do we make the extra effort to dispense meaning with our medicine? Why have we decided to be a place of discovery and not just a place of recovery? Why do we study innovation in companies outside of healthcare more often than in companies inside healthcare? Why do we view our work as sacred? And why does everyone around here feel lucky to be a part of this place?

Asking "why?" is a path to greatness, and yet, despite all this, it is one of the most infrequently answered of all questions. Leaders pay far more attention to "who," "what," "when," "where," and "how" than they do to "why."

Why?

Maybe we think that if we just tell our employees what to do and how to do it, they will follow our directions without question. In the book *What Managers Say and What Employees Hear*, Gary identified five reasons why the "Just Tell 'Em" approach doesn't work. Let's reprise that thinking here.

> *Why doesn't this 'Just Tell 'Em' approach work? And why, after so many failed attempts, do leaders still use it?*

> *Let's examine the underlying assumption upon which the 'Just Tell 'Em' approach is based. First, it assumes that the front line employees have the context and background information they need to understand major changes in strategic direction. But they don't. Even managers, who have much more information, often confess that they don't understand what it all means.*

> *Second, it assumes that employees totally accept the decisions of their top executives. They don't. Especially after so many 'major' change efforts have come and gone.*

Third, it assumes that employees don't have valid ideas of their own about where the company should be going. They do. And while they may be forced to accept the conclusions of management, they will still draw their own conclusions and act accordingly.

Fourth, this approach assumes the change is basically an information issue and that if they just knew the reasons why it would be good to change, they would change. They won't. Ask any smoker or overweight person about the accuracy of this assumption. Change is as much about relationships, emotions, and gut feel as it is about facts.

The fifth and final reason is that this approach assumes that no so-called fluff or entertainment value is needed, because the subject matter is so important and the people presenting it so noteworthy, employees will pay attention even if it's boring. They won't. This flies in the face of that old saying that 'Great teaching is one-fourth preparation and three-fourths theatre.'

Zero for Five: that's a bad night in any sport, especially the sport of strategic change.

The Context Story

If "Just Tell 'Em" doesn't work, what will? The context story is a special kind of story that leaders can deploy in a number of ways to unleash powerful understanding and emotional greatness in their organizations.

"Why?" is a context question. It adds intention, insight, and interest to the "what" and "how" of any business. A context story, then, can take the form of an operating theme and declaration, an adventure story on organizational strategy, inspirational all-staff events focused on the "why," and corporate university programs focused on culture, to name just a few. But no matter the form, the purpose of context stories is to plant two vital understandings firmly in the minds and hearts of everyone associated with your enterprise: Why do we do what we do? And why are we who we are? Let's take a look at some examples of context stories at work.

A New Cancer Center at St. Helena

Lots of cancer centers are being built these days, but how many of them can legitimately be called *new*? Sure, the walls, paint, carpet, and furniture qualify, but what about the actual patient experience? Is it new or just a version of what came before? Could the multiple-episode nature of cancer treatments be transformed into a meaningful, even spiritual relationship? And could this relationship go beyond treating the disease to transforming the patient's life and healing the family? All of these questions, and many more, were swirling in the head of JoAline Olson, the president and CEO of the 181-bed St. Helena (CA) Hospital, as she contemplated the challenge of conceiving, funding, building, and operating a truly different program in the heart of Napa Valley. Where would the patients come from? Where would the money come from? Where would the doctors and the major medical center affiliations come from? Where would the innovations in patient experience and healing come from? It seemed nearly impossible.

Fast-forward five years. Olson is now vice president of innovation for Adventist Health, which comprises 18 hospitals, including St. Helena. The hospital has raised more than $27 million and has designed a new-to-the-world patient experience, complete with the operating theme and declaration, "Abundant Health. Abundant Hope. Abundant Healing." The Martin O'Neil Cancer Center is set to open in November 2009. How did all this happen? "We never let ourselves get distracted by what we lack, by the scarcity of the situation," Olson says. "We stayed focused on abundance; that made all the difference."

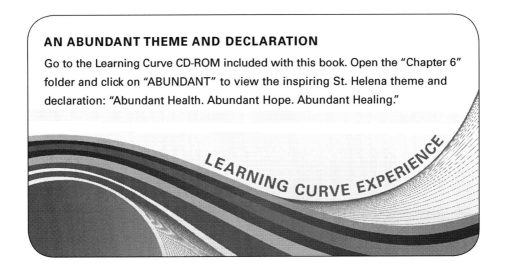

AN ABUNDANT THEME AND DECLARATION

Go to the Learning Curve CD-ROM included with this book. Open the "Chapter 6" folder and click on "ABUNDANT" to view the inspiring St. Helena theme and declaration: "Abundant Health. Abundant Hope. Abundant Healing."

LEARNING CURVE EXPERIENCE

As you can tell, "Abundant Health. Abundant Hope. Abundant Healing." gives context to the myriad important decisions that Olson and her team made along the way. Chances are that even if you'd never heard of the Martin O'Neil Cancer Center until today, you have a pretty clear idea of what it's like. That's the power of an operational theme and declaration. It answers the greatness question

"Why?" in a variety of important ways. Here are a few examples:

- Why did we change operation flow so that the patient can be seen in the cancer center the day of his or her diagnosis?

- Why did we establish a separate electronic link with family members so that they know precisely what to do to help?

- Why do we study the unique life circumstances of each patient apart from his or her disease?

- Why do we assign a Nurse Navigator and an Experience Guide to anticipate personal preferences and extend the relationship beyond the walls of the cancer center?

- Why did we design the facility as a healing environment and give every room an inspiring name, guided by our theme?

- And why did we hire nationally renowned artist Carol Jeanotilla to design a Hope Tree for the central atrium, complete with 48 Hope Symbols from around the world that staff members use when performing daily ceremonies for patients, families, and themselves?

These are just a handful of the many things that make this cancer center new in every sense of the word. And when it is consistently operated in accordance with the "Abundant Health. Abundant Hope. Abundant Healing." theme it won't only be new—it will be great.

A Driving Theme at Mid-Columbia Medical Center

A small place that has achieved big results is Mid-Columbia Medical Center (MCMC), a 50-bed hospital in The Dalles, OR. Much has been written about MCMC since it became the first hospital in the country to use the Planetree model systemwide. MCMC employs a three-word operating theme to guide and give context to everything it does: "Personalize. Humanize. Demystify." Leaders' unwavering dedication to use those three words to guide every decision enabled MCMC to accomplish things that were previously thought to be impossible in a hospital that size, such as drawing patients to the hospital from more than a dozen states, attracting renowned physicians from academic medical centers, and hosting thousands of site visits from all around the world so that others could study their innovations. As with most great companies, MCMC was not satisfied with its groundbreaking success. Leaders asked themselves what would happen if they applied their theme not only to the patient experience but also to the employee experience. The discoveries they made by doing this were truly remarkable.

> **RAIDERS OF THE LOST ART**
>
> Please return to the Learning Curve CD-ROM included with this book. Open the "Chapter 6" folder and click on "ART" to see how MCMC adapted an adventure story called "Raiders of the Lost Art" to immerse its employees in the new strategy and how it built a themed "corporate university" space to carry the context to new heights that included an award for the best corporate university among all Planetree hospitals.
>
> *LEARNING* CURVE EXPERIENCE

The Power of Context at Sharp HealthCare

Sharp has used the power of context stories most notably in its annual All-Staff Assemblies and the culture-oriented programs taught through The Sharp University. Sharp HealthCare's all-staff event started as a unique and bold method to set forth a new vision for the organization and to rally the entire workforce to become architects of change. Originally conceived as a recommitment ceremony, the event blended the power of story and ceremony to connect the hearts and minds of the organization's team members in a way that would drive individual and collective action and dramatic change. The All-Staff Assembly would be the first time the entire Sharp HealthCare team (a team the size of some small cities) would have the opportunity to collectively meet and hear from President and CEO Michael W. Murphy.

Murphy created context for the organization through story. Authentic, heartfelt stories and anecdotes culled from letters and real-life experiences. Stories that sparked laughter. And stories that sparked tears. Stories that reconnected the Sharp team to the purpose of their work and the noble difference team members make in the lives of those they serve. Stories that illuminated the difference between what Sharp HealthCare was and what Sharp HealthCare could and should be.

The first assembly brought to life not only what could be done to transform the healthcare experience for staff members and patients, but also why change and a better experience for patients was of critical importance. And why we were the people to make it happen. It was this connection to heart and purpose that excited and engaged the Sharp team and unleashed the momentum that has come to be known as The Sharp Experience and that continues to grow each year. The assembly has evolved into Sharp's signature employee engagement event: using the power of story to create context on many different levels via a variety of unique methods.

Event theme, invitations, and venue tell a story and can help to inform and provide context. Each All-Staff Assembly is themed to align to the overarching vision of the organization and the role each team member plays in achieving that vision, including the following:

Greetings and partings

Just as the simple acts of greetings and goodbyes make a difference in the experiences we create for our patients and guests, that notion is extended to the All-Staff Assembly to confirm the importance of warm welcomes and fond farewells. When we craft these touch points to be stories in and of themselves, they add to the experience for our team members and spark the telling of stories by team members about the event and the organization.

An army of greeters, including the entire executive leadership team, don event attire, grab a plastic hand "clapper," and form a human greeting tunnel to welcome and cheer the workforce as the heroes of Sharp's story. There's really nothing quite like it. In fact, many team members "run the tunnel" over and over again because it is such an uplifting experience. Additionally, a choir comprising physicians and caregivers from across the organization rehearses for three months in advance of the event. They perform as a way to honor, celebrate, and welcome the workforce to the assembly. Of course, the song is aligned to theme and purpose and, through music, tells a piece of the story. When it's time to say goodbye, team members receive a fond farewell and a musical escort to their awaiting buses—complete with high-fives, confetti, or other memorable moments.

CEO as storyteller

What could be construed as a traditional business update from the organization's CEO provides the best of both worlds: the business-critical content that aligns each employee to the goals of the organization, along with a vibrant use of story to bring meaning to the information. Organizational report card information is depicted through staff or physician personal narratives, the reading of letters or notes, video testimonials, or theatrical elements to punctuate a key point.

Due recognition

"Team Member Success" is a component of the event during which Sharp team members share their personal success stories related to their unique skill and success with a particular fundamental element of The Sharp Experience. When peers provide a context story, they help people make positive connections to their own work and life.

Personal stories

The powerful and personal stories of patients, physicians, and staff members are brought to life through both comprehensive documentary video and in-person participation. When we invite our patients and caregivers to share their stories with us, we have a direct connection to the purpose and why of our work. Read more about personal stories in Chapter 7.

Awards and accolades

Recognizing team members for individual, department, or team success aligned to the vision of the organization allows for details and stories to be told that enliven those who go above and beyond and help to paint a picture of why it matters. Sharp HealthCare's highest honors, known as the Pillars of Excellence awards, are bestowed at the assembly each year. The awards were created by team members from across the organization focused on enhancing the employee experience through reward and recognition. So the award process each year provides the opportunity to tell the story of how the awards were born—by the people, for the people—and also tell the story of the 18 award recipients.

Expert story time

Guest speakers are invited to share their story to provide inspiration and education to the Sharp team. Outside speakers provide an interesting dimension and help to shed new light for our journey. At Sharp, speakers are selected specifically for their ability to share their personal story—with the focus on the difference one human being can make in the lives of others. The connection that team members have made between The Sharp Experience and guest speaker stories has been astounding. These unique connections helped us to better understand that The Sharp Experience is really about helping our team members become better people, better parents, and better citizens. And through their personal growth, they become better team members and better leaders. This makes the why of our work all the more meaningful.

Work can be fun

Creating core components that are lighthearted and fun ensures that team members understand that although the work we do is serious, we can find time for fun and enjoy our colleagues through communal laughter and celebration. Whether it's the executive team honoring the organization through a hilarious dance number or a spoof of music videos aligned to a theme, building in elements of fun ensures a positive experience and a deeper understanding of what it takes to craft a transformational experience.

Story gathering

The All-Staff Assembly uses the rich stories of the people of Sharp HealthCare to help rally the organization to a brighter future: stories that convey our history (who we were), our present (who we are), and the need to become something more (who we could and should be). The event is a perfect venue to tap into and collect new stories from across the organization. Various interactive techniques are used to capture stories for future use, including video testimonials, interactive walls with key prompts, writing stations, and the distribution of personal journals for team members to capture their stories in the moment.

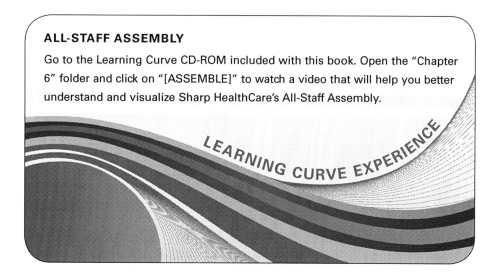

ALL-STAFF ASSEMBLY

Go to the Learning Curve CD-ROM included with this book. Open the "Chapter 6" folder and click on "[ASSEMBLE]" to watch a video that will help you better understand and visualize Sharp HealthCare's All-Staff Assembly.

LEARNING CURVE EXPERIENCE

Reflections

Although the All-Staff Assembly provides macro and micro opportunities for providing context through story, limiting story to just an annual event would be shortsighted. Storytelling is built into every aspect of The Sharp Experience as a way to keep the momentum going. In addition to grand storytelling opportunities such as the All-Staff Assembly, all gatherings at Sharp—large or small—begin with what Sharp calls a reflection: a story, quote, or letter that connects to the purpose of the work and helps focus on the importance of the task at hand. By taking a few moments at the beginning of every meeting to engage the hearts of our team members and reconnect to the why of our work, we fan the flames of enthusiasm and enlist our team members to share their spark of possibility.

When we connect the heart and the head of our team members and provide context and meaning to the work they do, we unleash the potential for truly extraordinary experiences. As healthcare leaders, how you choose to use story to convey why you do what you do will forever change the stories that are told in your organization, about your organization, and throughout the entire healthcare industry.

GARY'S STORY

In the 30 years I've been a consultant, I have repeatedly observed something very disappointing about the field: Consultants rarely do in their own business what they advise clients to do in theirs. This practice, or, should I say, lack of practice, is so common that consultants are mocked by their clients with almost the same frequency as lawyers. (One television ad featured a CEO who gave his consultant a directive to "Do it," to which the consultant replies with surprise and disdain: "We don't do what we advise. We just advise it.")

When I was conceiving Starizon as a new-to-the-world experience design and staging business, it seemed obvious to me that I should challenge the conventional wisdom in my industry to the same degree I would be asking clients to do in theirs. Further, I should design Starizon as a staged experience and not a tradition-bound delivered service. Although this all made great sense to me, it was nonsense to my consulting colleagues, as Joe Pine pointed out in the Foreword of this book. One of my "friends" in the business went so far as to make a list of 26 reasons that Starizon, as described in the business plan, couldn't possibly succeed. The things he said were impossible, or at the very least ill advised, included making consulting a multisensory experience, teaching clients all of our trade secrets, building an immersive experience place that clients would willingly travel to, not billing by the hour but instead allowing our clients to determine what the work was worth, casting our clients as explorers, and even having some famous explorers "show up" at Starizon to teach important lessons.

When he saw that his list didn't discourage me, he threw this in as number 26: "And what's with the name, anyway? Star-starvation?" Although I thought his word play was clever, I'm glad I didn't listen to the rest of his list. I'm glad I have taken every bit of the advice Sonia and I are offering to you in this book and applied it in my own business. I'm glad that Starizon answered the greatness question "Why?" through an operating theme and declaration. And I'm glad that for a decade, we've acted as though every decision we make is either a deposit or a withdrawal from the bank account of trust and meaning described in our declaration. But by far, I am most glad about what our clients have written and said about how Starizon has transformed their companies and lives.

Just think, if I can do all that with the mundane field of consulting, imagine what you can do with the vibrant field of healthcare.

LEARNING CURVE EXPERIENCE: GREETINGS FROM COLORADO

If you want to get an idea of what a theme, a declaration, and a place can do to transform the business-to-business experience of consulting, go to the Learning Curve CD-ROM, open the Chapter 6 folder, click on "DECLARE" and listen to the "Explore. Discover. Transform." declaration and take a visual tour of Starizon's Keystone, CO, home.

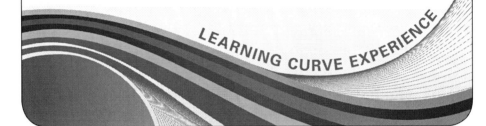

LEARNING CURVE EXPERIENCE

 The Complete Guide to Transforming the Patient Experience

LIVING LEGENDS:
Bringing Mission, Vision, and Values to Life

Why is it that after months of careful crafting and thoughtful review to make sure it's just right, the mission, vision, and values statements of most healthcare organizations don't make much of an operational impact? Is it because they try to cover too many things and thereby dissipate their effect? Sometimes. Is it that they are perceived as statements of intention and not requirements of action? Often. But the real problem is a lack of stories that bring the words to life. You must collect stories that offer genuine evidence and emotional proof that the mission, vision, and values are already being lived throughout the organization—ones that show concretely what it feels like when that happens.

The Power of Personal Stories

The best way to do this is through what we call "personal stories." They are the lifeblood of vibrant organizations. They address, head-on, the fact that most employees think management is much more interested in identifying and fixing what's wrong than celebrating and expanding what's right. This unfortunate reality is understandable when you consider there are many more courses in the average business school curriculum on problem solving than on storytelling. Many of our problems would solve themselves if only we did a better job of showing what our extraordinary performers are already doing. But instead of devoting the effort and attention it takes to expand the impact of our best people beyond the areas they work in every day, we devote it to trying to intervene with our worst people and change them into what they don't want to become. Like Sisyphus, we continue to try to roll these rocks up the hill, only to find that they continue to seek the bottom. We need to focus on those who strive to reach the pinnacle—and stay there! If our organizations are to become great, we must focus on the greatness that already exists within them. We must create living legends.

Personal stories can do just that.

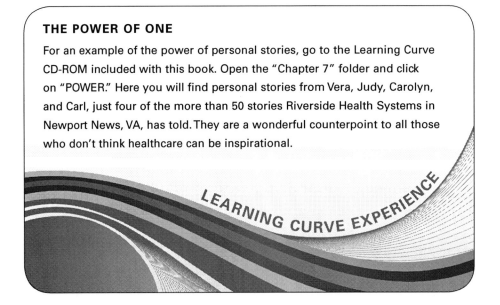

THE POWER OF ONE

For an example of the power of personal stories, go to the Learning Curve CD-ROM included with this book. Open the "Chapter 7" folder and click on "POWER." Here you will find personal stories from Vera, Judy, Carolyn, and Carl, just four of the more than 50 stories Riverside Health Systems in Newport News, VA, has told. They are a wonderful counterpoint to all those who don't think healthcare can be inspirational.

LEARNING CURVE EXPERIENCE

       The Complete Guide to Transforming the Patient Experience

What effect do you think the stories from Vera, Judy, Carolyn, Carl, and others have in the community? On the Riverside brand? On everyone who works at Riverside? On the people who the stories are about? The effect is exponential.

Sharp, too, has used personal stories in powerful ways. Let's build off our belief that transforming the healthcare experience for patients and customers requires a focus and commitment to transforming the healthcare experience for employees and physicians. And that only by focusing on creating the very best caregiver experience can a new-to-the-world patient experience emerge and sustain. So it is with personal stories. When we put forth new tools, skills, and behaviors for our team members to use as they create new experiences for our patients, it is vital that we intentionally seek out and catch our star performers in action as they bring the values and vision to life through the consistent use of these tools, skills, and behaviors. That which gets recognized most definitely gets repeated. So catching our top talent in the act and intentionally sharing stories and examples of team members going above and beyond articulates the importance and value of these behaviors far more than any memo ever would. These team member stories, when repeated, develop into corporate folklore—stories that are told over and over— that ultimately become part of the DNA of an organization.

I'll Take You There

When Sharp HealthCare launched The Sharp Experience in 2001 with a vision to transform the healthcare experience and make Sharp the best place to work, practice medicine, and receive care, the leadership engaged Sharp team members in envisioning the core standards of behavior for everyone. The 12 standards of behavior were introduced to the workforce with the expectation that team members would use them to guide their actions every day. Although the behaviors consisted of simple, basic actions, the challenge was to ensure that Sharp's 14,000 team members exhibited these behaviors with every interaction. One of the behaviors was specific to escorting patients and guests to their destination in Sharp facilities, rather than pointing or giving directions, thereby enlisting team members to use a "let me take you there" philosophy.

Hospitals and medical clinics can be confusing to navigate, and escorting patients and guests to their destination would allow for a far more personal interaction and experience. Stories began to emerge immediately—patients touched by the personal attention provided or unexpected reunions of long lost friends. One truly memorable story took place on a weekend at Sharp's corporate offices. The offices house traditional business support services, and no healthcare services are rendered at the corporate facility. President and CEO Mike Murphy, who is known for working on Saturday mornings, left the corporate office just after noon. As he walked out the front door, he ran into a family attempting to find a way into the building (the offices are locked on the weekends). Murphy asked if he could help them and they told him they had just learned that a family member was in Sharp Memorial Hospital, about 2 miles away. They had used an online mapping service that misdirected them to the corporate office. Murphy, who was wearing casual weekend attire, told the family that the hospital was a couple of miles down the road. For a split second he considered providing them directions, but quickly thought better of it. "At Sharp, we like to take people where they are going," he said. "Let me get my car, and you can follow me to the hospital." Others working at the corporate office that day saw what transpired. The story of Mike Murphy escorting family members to the hospital has become legendary.

Telling stories of team members embodying the tenets of The Sharp Experience is now part of who Sharp is as an organization. These stories are often used as reflections at the beginning of meetings and are conveyed through employee forums, new employee orientation, internal magazines, the employee intranet, and face to face. In the early days of The Sharp Experience, these stories created tremendous excitement; the thought that these new behaviors were making a difference confirmed that Sharp was on the right path. As the stories began to proliferate, the Sharp team, along with its advertising agency, thought it could be interesting to bring a video crew into the facilities to catch people in the act or to have them share their own personal stories of The Sharp Experience on camera. The idea was to film, documentary style, with the hope that the footage could be used as a story-telling mechanism at the next All-Staff Assembly. It took only a few hours of footage in Sharp facilities to realize that the stories unfolding every day with caregivers and patients should be told beyond the doors of Sharp HealthCare. Very quickly, a strategy was developed to create a 30-minute television documentary featuring the stories of Sharp staff members, physicians, and patients. This 30-minute documentary, called "Stories of the Sharp Experience," became the centerpiece of an entirely new marketing strategy and campaign. Using its people and patients as story-tellers in an unscripted, unrehearsed, authentic look at the dedication of the entire team to make healthcare better, Sharp was able to share the story with the community and begin to differentiate the organization in the marketplace.

The documentary chronicles compelling patient stories along with unique depictions of the unsung healthcare heroes at Sharp, working diligently to make The Sharp Experience a reality. From the dramatic story of a pregnant woman who was hit by a car at a bus stop and who underwent surgery that saved both her and her baby to the sweet story of a hospital chef who is passionate about doing his part for staff members and patients, the documentary provides the community with a clear understanding of the journey the organization is on to improve the healthcare experience. And although sharing these in-depth stories with the community sets Sharp up for possible criticism from those who might insist "That's not the experience I had at Sharp," it also holds the organization accountable for continuing the quest to create healthcare the way it was meant to be. Sharing stories of The Sharp Experience with the community makes it much harder to lose focus or give up when times are tough.

The reality-style documentary transformed Sharp's traditional advertising into a new storytelling platform. The 30-minute documentary served as the signature of a campaign that included 60- and 30-second television commercials and 60-second radio advertisements. Since 2002, the Sharp team has produced seven annual 30-minute documentaries and complementary call-to-action commercials. Each year, the documentary is aired more than 150 times on local and cable television stations along with aligned 60- and 30-second television and radio commercials.

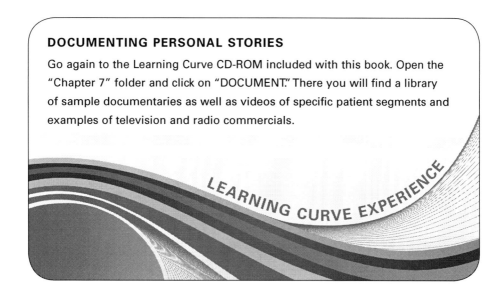

DOCUMENTING PERSONAL STORIES

Go again to the Learning Curve CD-ROM included with this book. Open the "Chapter 7" folder and click on "DOCUMENT." There you will find a library of sample documentaries as well as videos of specific patient segments and examples of television and radio commercials.

LEARNING CURVE EXPERIENCE

The Story Premiers

As we've learned from Joe Pine and Jim Gilmore, the new consumer sensibility is authenticity. Not only are consumers seeking positively memorable experiences, but they also must perceive those experiences as real. Sharp takes this understanding of authenticity to heart. All Sharp advertising and marketing feature only the real people and real stories of Sharp. No actors, no models. Not glossy, not perfect.

Each year, the television documentary is premiered at the All-Staff Assembly before airing for the community. The show and stories are seen as a gift to the organization and a gift to the community. A truly memorable feature of the All-Staff Assembly is when the staff, physicians, and patients featured in the show are invited on stage and honored by the Sharp team. These patients are brave and giving to share their personal healthcare journey with the world. It's so uplifting for the organization to cheer for these patients—many whom have been through unbeliev-able circumstances. Attendees will never forget watching a 19-year-old boy walk across the stage at the assembly even though he was never supposed to walk again after a devastating spinal injury. Or the elderly gentleman basking in the glow of a standing ovation—his family by his side—after recovering from a catastrophic stroke. And truly memorable was the young woman being kept alive through a mechanical circulatory support device (also known as a left ventricular assist device) who found out the day of the assembly that she was now eligible for a heart transplant. She shared her good news with Sharp's 14,000 team members, who erupted in ecstatic support for her. Not long after her experience at the All-Staff Assembly, she stated that she originally was nervous about the thought of a heart transplant, but with the overwhelming support of the 14,000 people of Sharp, she knew she could go through with it.

Finding the Stories

Leaders have to become versed in both storytelling and story gathering. Processes and mechanisms should be in place to make it easy and natural. Rather than add cumbersome steps or processes for gathering stories, Sharp capitalizes on existing mechanisms such as leader rounding and thank-you notes to collect and share positive stories. Leaders use a prescribed process to round on their direct reports, physicians, and patients, and they use a rounding log as an aid to document what's working well, what's getting in the way, and any positive stories that could and should be shared. This way, every single day Sharp leaders are collecting stories throughout the organization.

    The Complete Guide to Transforming the Patient Experience

Sharp also uses rounding as a way to identify team members who go above and beyond. Those team members then receive a handwritten thank-you note from their boss, or better yet, their boss' boss. Thank-you notes are sent to the homes of these deserving employees, and the notes have taken on a life of their own. Team members have been so moved by receiving a thank-you note, they share them with their friends and families, post them on their refrigerators or their office wall at work, and will talk about and remember them forever. Some Sharp leaders are known for sending handwritten thank-you notes to the children of their employees. These notes are typically sent when a team member has put in long hours working on an important project. When the kids get a note that says "Thank you for sharing your mom with us at Sharp HealthCare. She's an incredible member of our team," there's a "wow" and a lot of storytelling. Not long after one team member's children received a note like this, she brought the kids to the office to meet her boss. She thanked her boss for helping her serve as a positive role model for her children. Talk about "wow"!

Sharp's attitude of gratitude spread like wildfire, and before long, staff members began sending handwritten thank-you notes to the homes of patients, thanking them for trusting Sharp with their care. Sharp leaders were not aware of this new practice and found out only because patients started sending thank-you notes for the thank-you notes. Notes to patients are signed by all caregivers and say "Thank you for trusting us with your healthcare. It was an honor caring for you." These notes to patients sparked stories across the community. Patients would tell their friends about the note and many would bring the note into a follow-up meeting with their physician. Physicians wanted to get into the act and asked whether they too could sign the notes that were sent when a patient was discharged from the hospital. One patient even wrote to the *San Diego Union Tribune* about the note he received after a hospital visit, and the newspaper then wrote an article about the note. There has been a ripple of gratitude across the organization and community and a rich source of stories to gather and share. Every interaction is an opportunity to find or tell a story. And when your patients begin telling your story for you, you know you're on the right track.

Not All Stories Are Good Stories

Context stories and personal stories can align, engage, and excite your team members. Connecting team members to the purpose of their work and the difference they make through these inspiring stories can create a positive self-fulfilling prophecy. Wouldn't it be great if all healthcare stories were positive? The more we do to create exceptional healthcare experiences, the more likely we are to see positive healthcare stories. But the reality is that the media rarely covers a positive healthcare story, and consumers, all too often, are exposed only to the scary stories of mistakes or problems in healthcare. We can use these less-than-positive stories to move the organization forward as well.

When a patient at Sharp had the perfect storm of experiences (you know the kind—when everything that can go wrong does go wrong), Sharp took the opportunity to learn from this patient's story. The patient was invited to share his story at a Quarterly Leadership Development Session (sessions created to develop the 1,400 leaders at Sharp). This gentleman took the stage and began his story by saying,

 The Complete Guide to Transforming the Patient Experience

"I'm here to share the story of my Sharp Experience—and it's a Sharp Experience of a different kind."

He proceeded to share the details of his multiple experiences with the organization. Experiences that unfortunately and unintentionally robbed him of his dignity and experiences that changed his health and his life. He spoke for nearly an hour to a perfectly still and hushed room. The only sounds were the stifled sniffles and sobs from the audience as they listened to his story. When he ended his story, the room was raw. But the room was also appreciative. Leaders lined up at microphones to ask questions and make comments. Through tears, they told him how sorry they were for his experience. The entire leadership team made commitments to ensure that no one else would experience what he had experienced. The patient told the group that his purpose in sharing his story was to do what he could to keep others from having the same experience. He was giving Sharp a gift by sharing his story—a gift that would help the organization to learn and grow. As a result, teams were formed to address the concerns, and immediate improvements were put in place. This one negative story helped to create incredible positive change. And it helped the entire organization better understand the "why."

Are You Open to Stories?

We are so fortunate to work in healthcare, an industry ripe with opportunities to make a difference. Our team members, patients, and guests will always have a story to share if we are open and willing to hear it. Being open means using every chance you have to connect in a meaningful way with another human being. When we live our life "heads up, eyes up, and smiles on," we are an invitation to others to engage. Our patients and guests are often in our facilities unexpectedly and are living through some of the most challenging experiences of their lives. The simple act of walking through the halls with the purposeful intention of connecting—of being there for others—makes all the difference. When we look people in the eye, smile, and say "good afternoon," you can see in an instant whether someone is lost, hurting, or in need. Take those opportunities to ask whether you may be of assistance. You never know how needed you really are unless you ask. Here's an example.

SONIA'S STORY

Not long ago, I was asked to speak at a hospital in another community about the Sharp experience. While there, I behaved as I always do—head up, eyes up, smile on—engaging each person I encountered with a "good morning" and an offer of assistance. It quickly became obvious that this was not the normal behavior for this hospital, because people began to stop me for directions and ask for my assistance (although I didn't observe that happening with any of the actual employees of that hospital also walking through the halls). Mind you, I was not wearing a uniform or a badge from this hospital—I simply engaged those I passed in the hall. After giving a keynote presentation for some hospital leaders, I went to lunch in the cafeteria with a hospital executive. I greeted everyone I encountered, and said "good afternoon" to a lovely older woman at the table next to me, making small talk. The woman excitedly talked about the food items on her tray—French fries and onion rings. She mentioned that she didn't usually eat fries and rings, but that she was celebrating. I was eager to know what the celebration was and asked her to share it with me. The lovely woman, with glistening eyes, grabbed my hand and told me that she had just received news that she was now five years free of cancer and that she had been given a clean bill of health.

Good news is meant to be shared, and this woman was simply waiting for someone to give her the opportunity to share her story. For me, it was a highlight of my week. How fortunate to be the first person to hear this incredible news!

Everyone has a story. Take time to tell stories, gather stories, and be open to unexpected stories. There are useful techniques that can ensure that your personal stories are powerful and connected to your mission, vision, and values.

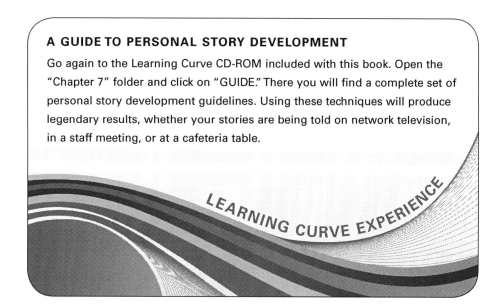

A GUIDE TO PERSONAL STORY DEVELOPMENT

Go again to the Learning Curve CD-ROM included with this book. Open the "Chapter 7" folder and click on "GUIDE." There you will find a complete set of personal story development guidelines. Using these techniques will produce legendary results, whether your stories are being told on network television, in a staff meeting, or at a cafeteria table.

MINIATURE TREASURES, EPIC RESULTS:
Celebration Ceremonies and Signature Moments

Now that you have two arrows in your storytelling quiver, context stories, and personal stories, let's look at how celebration ceremonies and signature moments can reshape the trajectory of the brand promise and, more importantly, the brand experience in your company. Together they are a powerful story form.

The Whole Experience in Miniature

Ceremonies, whether they're performed as celebrations for staff members or as signature moments for patients and families, remind us that nothing is insignificant in the story of our organizations. As they say at Disney, "everything speaks;" it's just a question of whether it speaks intentionally and inspirationally or haphazardly and hollowly. Mother Teresa said it best: "We do no great things. Only small things with great love." And when we do enough small things with great love, we will have established a set of rich traditions that are the hallmarks of every truly great place.

The great thing about ceremonies is that they take the whole of the experience and recast it as a memorable set of miniature treasures.

A woman named Mary

Mark Scott, the former CEO at Mid-Columbia Medical Center (MCMC) who is now a Starizon partner, thinks that most of the extraordinary progress his team made in transforming healthcare can be attributed to storytelling. His manager retreats told stories. His physical spaces—both remodeled and brand new—told stories. Before each meeting, participants told stories that were examples of values and excellence at work at MCMC. These stories were collected as the most important part of the minutes. There were ceremonial celebrations of all shapes and sizes, each with a special memento. But for all the story-laden ceremonies Mark performed for others, one that was performed for him may best illustrate their power.

Mark was the only healthcare CEO invited to the Service Quality Leadership Forum. The purpose of the forum, which met for several years in the early 1990s, was to unite CEOs from leading companies in a variety of industries in the quest to understand what it takes to create a vibrant, turned-on, high-performing company. In other words, what it takes to make greatness. They studied each other's progress and failures. They gleaned great insights and forged strong relationships. One of the people Mark particularly connected with was Mary. She had been one of the first women in the United States to rise to the level of senior management as the national training director for a large direct-sale business.

Although her success in both places was great, something caused her to leave the world of big business and start her own company. You see, far too often when

Mary was in a top executive meeting and proposed an unusually creative idea, her male colleagues would scoff and say, "Mary, there you go again—you're thinking like a woman." As you can imagine, this cut her to the core—so much so that she went out and established a company that has produced more women millionaires than any other on the planet. Her name was Mary Kay Ash, and her story is known far beyond the halls of the cosmetics company she built. Well, Mary asked Mark to present his healthcare innovations at a meeting of several thousand of her sales associates. After he was done and the applause had died down, she joined him onstage and thanked him for all he and his team had done for healthcare. Then she presented him with the company's most valued award: a 50-cent pink button with the following inscription: "Thinking Like a Woman." It is one of Mark's most prized possessions.

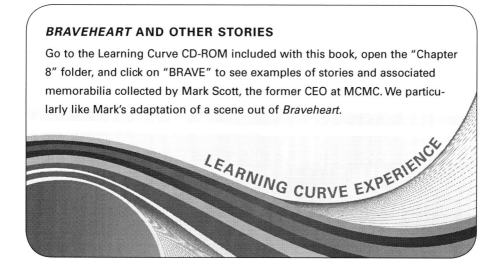

BRAVEHEART AND OTHER STORIES

Go to the Learning Curve CD-ROM included with this book, open the "Chapter 8" folder, and click on "BRAVE" to see examples of stories and associated memorabilia collected by Mark Scott, the former CEO at MCMC. We particularly like Mark's adaptation of a scene out of *Braveheart*.

LEARNING CURVE EXPERIENCE

An inviting structure

Ceremonies elevate the importance of small, everyday activities. They make the mundane memorable. The staircase at the College Football Hall of Fame in South Bend, IN, is a good example. The Hall of Fame is a two-story building, with the first story below ground. You walk in, purchase your tickets, and head toward the spiral staircase that takes you to the below-ground galleries, stadium, and interactive displays. If the designers had only concerned themselves with the functional aspects of getting from the second floor entry to the first floor displays, they would have missed a huge storytelling opportunity. Fortunately, they decided to support the story structure of the building, not just its physical structure.

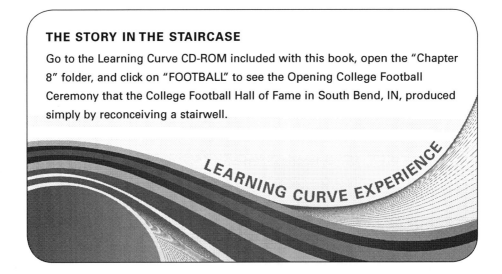

THE STORY IN THE STAIRCASE

Go to the Learning Curve CD-ROM included with this book, open the "Chapter 8" folder, and click on "FOOTBALL" to see the Opening College Football Ceremony that the College Football Hall of Fame in South Bend, IN, produced simply by reconceiving a stairwell.

LEARNING CURVE EXPERIENCE

There is a two-story-tall sculpture of all things college football: players, equipment, play diagrams, books, lockers, Gatorade, even pizza boxes. The stair ramp winds around the sculpture as it descends to the lower level so that you can take in the power of this monument from all different angles. But that's not all. At periodic

 The Complete Guide to Transforming the Patient Experience

stopping points on the ramp are inspirational passages from Charlie Loftus' great book *What is a Football Player?* So you are seeing the images and reading the words at the same time, just as you would with a good storybook. But even that's not all, because then they make the images move. On a series of TV screens embedded around the sculpture are short video vignettes of a kid who grows up to be a college football player. You see him learning how to pass and catch with his dad in the backyard. Then you see him playing pee-wee football, then high school football, and finally achieving his dream of playing in college. You find yourself emotionally engaged. It makes you believe that college football must be the greatest thing ever invented. And all you've done is walk down the ramp from the second floor entrance to the first floor exhibits. It is a magnificent opening ceremony that performs itself for every person who enters the Hall of Fame. And after you have spent several hours downstairs, guess what? You leave the same way you came in, and a closing ceremony with added context is "reperformed" just for you. It's brilliant: an entry stairwell as a ceremony. How could you create a storytelling opening ceremony at an employee entrance or a hallway or an elevator lobby?

Ceremonies and symbols help to create story and memory out of what may otherwise be experienced as routine business. Take, for example, an organization's goals. How many employees are able to articulate the specific goals of an organization and understand the purpose and meaning behind them? Not nearly enough. If an organization is serious about significant change, and the key to that change is an engaged and aligned workforce, they must paint a memorable picture or craft a meaningful story to help team members understand and remember the goals and their part in achieving them.

A signing ceremony that seals commitment

When Sharp HealthCare set out to create a new-to-the-world healthcare experience, it created a new vision, a new structure, and a new model for change. That was a lot for the organization to comprehend in a short period of time. So it used ceremony and symbols to help excite and inspire employees and to better connect the dots from overarching organizational elements to the specific role of each team member. Sharp had adopted the Pillars of Excellence framework and many fundamentals from the Studer Group and aligned the organization by six pillars of excellence: quality, service, people, finance, growth, and community. The pillar framework simplified the aims of the organization and used easy-to-understand language and descriptions for the organizational goals under each pillar. The Sharp Experience initiative, the new vision, new framework, and new structure were first introduced to the organization's leaders and then to the entire workforce at the All-Staff Assembly. When leaders were brought together for their first immersion into the tenets of The Sharp Experience, they learned about the Pillars of Excellence and then were asked to sign their commitment to the Pillars of Excellence. The signing ceremony was filled with great pomp and circumstance as leaders selected which pillar to sign and where to place their name.

The signed pillars now stand in the lobby of Sharp HealthCare's corporate offices and serve as a symbol of every leader's commitment to The Sharp Experience. Along with the ceremonial signing of the pillars, a symbol was also introduced with the launch of The Sharp Experience. Sharp HealthCare adopted a flame as the symbol to represent The Sharp Experience endeavor. The flame stands for the fire and passion inside each individual and the fact that The Sharp Experience was

FIGURE 8.1

SIX PILLARS OF EXCELLENCE

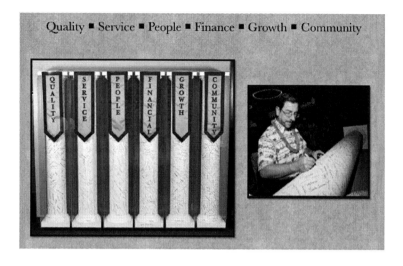

about sharing our spark of possibility with others, while fanning the flames of enthusiasm. The flame was included in The Sharp Experience logo and is easily recognized and understood by the entire organization.

When you have a symbol that is recognized and understood by all, there is so much more you can do to bring that symbol to life. The flame is incorporated into printed material in fun and creative ways, and a library of "fire" music to accompany key events, such as Johnny Cash's "Ring of Fire," "Light the Fire Within" by Leann Rimes, and "Keep the Fire Burnin' " by REO Speedwagon, serves as the soundtrack to The Sharp Experience. Sharp's CEO has been known to dress in a wild flame shirt, and events have included fire dancers to ensure that Sharp team members are "fired up."

The pillar and flame symbols are also used to provide reward and recognition for the Sharp team. The highest accolades for the organization take the form of Pillar of Excellence awards. (Recipients receive a handcrafted pillar statuette.) To be considered for a Pillar award, individuals, departments, and teams must first be recognized with a Center of Recognized Excellence, or CORE award, for their particular facility. The CORE awards represent the blue core or hot center of a flame. (The award is a blue acrylic flame.)

A helping hand for newcomers

New employees to Sharp are introduced to symbols and ceremony on their first day of work. At New Employee Orientation, every new employee receives a puffy, yellow "helping hand" sticker to affix to his or her new badge. The helping hand sticker serves as a symbol that makes it easy for other employees to quickly recognize that the employee is new and might need a helping hand. Employees know that when they encounter someone with a helping hand, they should introduce themselves and offer to be of assistance to the new team member. At the conclusion of the 90-day introductory period, new employees are invited, with their supervisor, to a special 90-day ceremony where each new employee is asked to share a positive story about his or her first three months and also identify opportunities for improvement for the organization. These moving stories are often about a personal, memorable encounter related to the helping hand sticker. At the 90-day ceremony, new employees pose for a group photo and then remove their helping hand sticker and place it alongside their photo. These photos are framed and displayed for all to see.

The power and importance of ceremony and symbols were brought to life when Sharp learned that new employees did not want to relinquish their helping hand sticker at the 90-day ceremony. They said they liked wearing the symbol and the interactions that the sticker sparked. As a result, a new blue helping hand sticker replaces the yellow sticker at the 90-day ceremony. This symbolizes the transition from needing a helping hand to becoming a helping hand for others.

Across the Sharp system, the use of ceremony has served as a meaningful and memorable method to help team members refuel, recharge, reenergize, reflect, and recommit.

An opening ceremony

At Sharp Coronado Hospital, the recent renovation of the second-floor Medical Surgical Patient Care Unit provided the opportunity for a very special staff ceremony. When the much-anticipated renovation was completed, all staff members participated in a welcome and recommitment ceremony.

Utilizing the shell motif that is found throughout this very unique boutique hospital on Coronado Island, the highlight of the ceremony was when team members selected a shell that they felt best represented them. They wrote their names on the shells and shared their personal commitment to the experience they create for each other and their patients.

One by one, these shells were placed in a glass urn. The shell-filled urn is now on display in the new second-floor great room and it serves as an elegant reminder of the special ceremony and personal commitments. It also serves as a meaningful prop and conversation-starter in the new great room in the unit that was designed to remove the traditional barriers between the nurses' stations and family waiting areas.

"The power of the recommitment ceremony for us was in each team member verbally sharing with others their heartfelt reasons for continuing their personal journey toward putting the patient first," said Marcia Hall, CEO of Sharp Coronado (CA) Hospital. "As each person, shy and otherwise, stepped up with their shell and their commitment, we could literally feel the team embracing their words, embracing their feelings. Everyone in the room was amplified and uplifted by the communal sense of being part of something very personal, yet bigger than each of us. I was moved and awestruck by the connection between heart and hands no matter if the team member was from housekeeping, engineering, or the operating room."

A quotable tradition

Ceremony provides a time and space for personal and collective connection and can take many different forms. What initially started as singular ceremonies have grown into long-standing, much-loved, rich traditions. Sharp's tradition of beginning meetings with a reflection has permeated every aspect of the organization. Team members are always at the ready with a story, quote, or saying. In fact, this tradition has spilled over into the décor of the brand-new Sharp Memorial Hospital. Key public spaces have meaningful, thought-provoking reflections painted across the walls.

The All-Staff Assembly has also evolved from a ceremony to a unique and lauded tradition. Initially conceived as a one-time recommitment ceremony—a time for Sharp's team members to recommit to the purpose of their work and the difference they make—it is now Sharp's signature employee engagement event with ceremony and tradition woven through each moment and aspect of the event. Transportation, greeting, welcoming, seating, participating, and departing all take on new meaning when designed as part of a special ceremony.

Ceremonies and Symbols to Wow Patients

Ceremonies and symbols enliven and enrich experiences and can also be used to create signature moments for our patients and guests. If the hallmark of an experience is a memory, a signature moment is a specific element of an experience that is intentionally designed to create a wow with our patients and guests and ensure a positively memorable experience. Signature moments can be thought of as the "experience within the experience," and at Sharp, every leader was immersed in the concepts of the experience economy and learned about signature moments. Each leader was then charged with identifying and creating a signature moment for his or her unit, department, or area of responsibility. When they were given the chance to serve as "memory makers," the creativity flowed as new Signature Moments were crafted and implemented.

Today, there are a wide variety of signature moments at Sharp and they are designed for both the team member experience and the patient/guest experience—and they are frequently updated or changed to ensure that they remain fresh. The following are just a few examples of Signature Moments at Sharp.

An angel among us

Sharp Coronado Hospital extends its beach/shell motif to a sweet signature moment for patients. A lovely staff nurse has taken to walking the beaches on her days off looking for a particular type of broken seashell that looks like an angel wing. The angel wings are given to patients, along with a meaningful quote, and patients can rub the angel wing when worried or nervous.

A refreshing touch

Sharp Coronado Hospital food service staff members created a signature moment for patients on the day they depart for home. They bake loaves of banana bread and wrap them in special Cellophane bags. A personalized card signed by the kitchen staff is tied to the package. Food service team members hand-deliver the banana bread to patients as they leave the hospital, letting them know it was "baked with love" so they would have a snack when they arrived safely at home.

An inspirational tradition

The admitting staff at Sharp Memorial Hospital felt disconnected from patients because of the business nature of their role. They created a completely new bedside registration experience, and along with making registration quick and easy right in the patient's room, they also come bearing an inspirational quote of the day for their patients. The admissions staff reads the quote to the patient and family, provides a printed copy for them, and tells them that they are happy to be part of their care team. The admissions staff then round each day on every patient they've personally admitted and provide a new inspirational quote of the day. Not only do patients enjoy the personal, inspirational experience, but the admissions staff members are also much more fulfilled in the work that they do.

     The Complete Guide to Transforming the Patient Experience

The silver tray treatment

The signature moment created for endoscopy patients at the Sharp Memorial Outpatient Pavilion is truly memorable. It's hard to believe, given that an endoscopy tends to be the one medical procedure that most people don't ever want to think about (an endoscopy is a procedure whereby a physician uses a special flexible scope to visualize the inside of the intestinal tract). Ensuring patient comfort and dignity is of utmost importance to the endoscopy team. To create a caring, memorable moment for patients after the procedure, staff members offer a special silver tray with juice in stemmed glassware, crackers, mints, and a warmed washcloth and hand towel.

Truly noteworthy

The thank-you notes that Sharp sends to the homes of patients serve as an organizationwide signature moment, not only eliciting "wows" from patients when they receive the notes, but also providing a "wow" for Sharp team members just by writing the notes. When team members write thank-you notes, they solidify a deep connection with their patients, which provides a further reminder of the purpose of their work. When patients receive thank-you notes, they better understand that Sharp HealthCare provides a different kind of healthcare experience.

When we take the time to conceive and perform celebration ceremonies and signature moments, we break the mold of healthcare the way it has always been and intentionally create a more meaningful, memorable healthcare experience for those who work in healthcare and those receiving their care in our facilities.

We make a statement that healthcare can be, and should be, inspirational. But perhaps most importantly, we take the whole of a very complex experience design and shrink it into something solid enough to hold in the palm of your hand and clear enough to be understood in the emotions of your heart: miniature treasures that create epic results.

STAGE DESIGN:
Turning Physical Structures into Story Structures

"It was the best of times. It was the worst of times."

The famous opening lines to Charles Dickens' *A Tale of Two Cities* could just as aptly describe the buildings in healthcare circa 2010 as the circumstances found in London and Paris circa 1775.

We are undergoing a true revolution in healthcare environments, where, for the first time in history, the buildings themselves are being conceived as instruments of healing. This is in stark contrast to the sterile, almost prison-like design ethic that ruled from the early days of hospital buildings. (The notable exception, as we discussed in Chapter 2, was maternity, which the baby boomers transformed starting in the early 1980s.) Although the functional ward has shrunk continuously from 64 beds to 32 to 16 to eight to four and finally to the current two-bed version that is now the standard, it has been the building block of choice.

The Best of Times

Many organizations—especially those that have begun the hard work of transforming the healthcare experience for their patients—are converting to all private rooms. But this is still far from the norm.

Steve Altmiller, former CEO of San Juan Regional Medical Center in Farmington, NM, discovered this when he received some surprising pushback to his proposal for an all-private-room hospital expansion. His answer to the skeptics who wanted to do things the same old way? "Of course we don't have to have all private rooms," he said. "We could recreate the semiprivate room design in our current hospital. But before we do that, I just need someone to show me the 'private part' of the semiprivate room." Of course, no one could do that, so Steve proposed a change in terminology. "I think we should call them what they really are: 'not-at-all-private rooms.'"

In storytelling, language is important. And the language Steve used to sway the skeptics worked: In the end, the expansion featured all private rooms and was a healing environment that few could have imagined would ever be built in the small town of Farmington.

Furthermore, the new hospital was infused with experiential details, including welcoming lobbies; a private outdoor balcony on each patient room; healing gardens; soothing lighting, colors, and textures; the sights, sounds, and smells of nature; personalized bedside technology; onstage and offstage facility design; and myriad other "small-is-beautiful," noninstitutional elements. Elements such as these have transformed, not merely improved, San Juan Regional.

The advantages of these new healing environments are tremendous. They can improve financial performance, clinical outcomes, and employee satisfaction and retention. Longitudinal studies, such as the Pebble Project developed by The Center for Health Design, document these and other benefits. When buildings are designed as healing instruments, surely it is the best of times in healthcare facilities.

The Worst of Times

And so it is the best of times, except for one tiny detail that's almost not worth mentioning, a detail that keeps people at the Concord, CA–based Center for Health Design and other places dedicated to the new healing environments movement up at night. After all this time, money, and expertise are spent in the design and construction of these new halls of healing, people invariably move in. And although that should not be a surprise, it often catches healthcare organizations unawares. Because when the move is not accompanied by a totally new patient experience concept that everybody thoroughly understands, along with comprehensive training and consistent reinforcement of the new patient experience concept, something else invariably happens: The old play is performed on the new stage. And nothing can be more damaging to the healing environment movement than performing the same impersonal, dehumanizing care in opulent surroundings. *Obnoxious* is the nicest word that comes to mind. When this happens, it is definitely the worst of times in healthcare facilities.

So concerned were the advocates of healing environments about this "expensive perfume on a pig" approach to the patient experience that they asked Gary to write a five-part series for the journal *Healthcare Design*, dedicated to an approach that changes the stage and the experience that is performed on it.

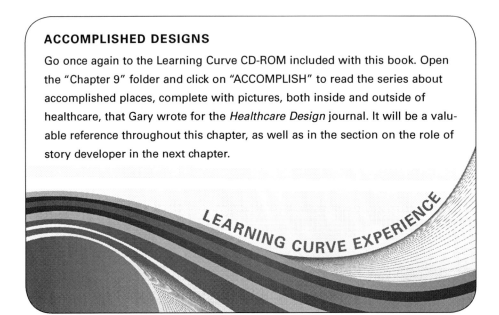

ACCOMPLISHED DESIGNS

Go once again to the Learning Curve CD-ROM included with this book. Open the "Chapter 9" folder and click on "ACCOMPLISH" to read the series about accomplished places, complete with pictures, both inside and outside of healthcare, that Gary wrote for the *Healthcare Design* journal. It will be a valuable reference throughout this chapter, as well as in the section on the role of story developer in the next chapter.

Story Structures

So what must we do to prevent turning the best of times in healthcare design into the worst of times? How can we get an experience ROI on the immense capital we are spending on new and remodeled stages? First, we must stop looking at these facilities as mere buildings, or just containers for the activities professionals carry out inside them. They are and should be much more than that. They are—excuse the pun—the most concrete and lasting way an organization tells its story. They are the interpretation of values, beliefs, and aspirations in stone and steel. They are "story structures." And if we conceive them as that, from the first block diagram through the logistics of the move-in process, we will avoid the disappointment of the new building being swallowed up by the old culture.

When we call our buildings "story structures," the language immediately changes our expectations. No longer are we guided only by traditional insights such as "form follows function." We can now augment this insight with the realization that in the experience economy, function must follow experience and that a great experience follows a storyline. This new design ethic (form follows function, function follows experience, and experience follows storyline) is much more than a change in semantics. It's a fundamental change in belief. Let's look at some examples of the design process based on this new belief.

A Bridge Beyond

We are fortunate to work with a group of ex-Disney "Imagineers," who collectively refer to themselves as the Spatial Stories Studio. They provide great insights in how to go beyond traditional architecture approaches to interpret a themed experience into a one-of-a-kind physical place. A great example of this work in healthcare is set in the rolling hills of Lancaster, PA.

Lancaster General Hospital sits at the crossroads of old and new. The old is the strong heritage of the Amish country in which it is located. The new is the increasing number of urban Philadelphia workers who live in the countryside of Lancaster County and commute into the city. Lancaster General's new North Campus must honor the traditional while also serving the progressive. It must also connect, in a more patient-centered way, the too often disjointed services and practitioners of medical care. And finally, Lancaster General wanted to link ill-ness treatment, health recovery, and wellness promotion in a seamless way.

You may have noticed that the elemental concept all these aspirations have in common is connection. If you were to visit this area of Pennsylvania, you might draw the conclusion that the book *The Bridges of Madison County* was written about the wrong place—it should have been called *The Bridges of Lancaster County*. There are trussed and covered bridges of all shapes, colors, and sizes. They connect one place with another and serve as an iconic story element for the connected version of healthcare that Lancaster General wants to build.

Using the theme "Building a Bridge Beyond" as the foundation of its story struc-tures, a team from Lancaster General and the Spatial Stories Studio rendered a captivating tale to be told in wood, steel, and glass.

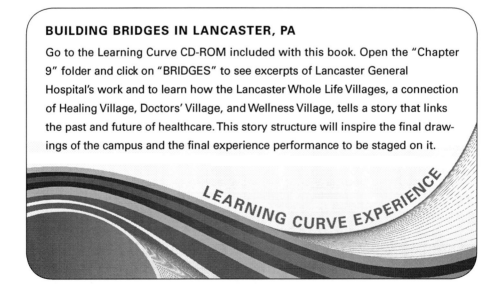

BUILDING BRIDGES IN LANCASTER, PA

Go to the Learning Curve CD-ROM included with this book. Open the "Chapter 9" folder and click on "BRIDGES" to see excerpts of Lancaster General Hospital's work and to learn how the Lancaster Whole Life Villages, a connection of Healing Village, Doctors' Village, and Wellness Village, tells a story that links the past and future of healthcare. This story structure will inspire the final draw-ings of the campus and the final experience performance to be staged on it.

LEARNING CURVE EXPERIENCE

     The Complete Guide to Transforming the Patient Experience

Inspiring by Design

Starizon's building in Keystone, CO, is another example of the story structure. It is a huge departure from the standard glass wall conference room surrounded by staff cubicles and windowed partner offices that is commonplace in the consulting industry. It is a destination that immerses clients in the tenets of experience design and staging, as well as their power to explore, discover, and transform themselves and their industries. Clients travel to Colorado to visit Starizon (turning on its head the conventional wisdom that clients would never travel to their consultants and that consultants must always instead visit clients). The spaces within are named "Aspire," "Invent," "Create," "Believe," and "Discover," to single out just a few. The names and the setting help set the tone for the special work that has happened there over the years.

Both Lancaster General's North Campus and Starizon share a very important advantage. They were conceived as story structures from the outset. But what do you do if you are remodeling an existing place? Or what if you're already well into the construction of a new building? Is it too late to employ the transforming power of story structures? Definitely not, as two examples from Sharp will now demonstrate.

The Nautilus Proportion

Sharp Coronado Hospital is the oldest and smallest of Sharp HealthCare's hospital facilities. Just 10 years ago, Sharp Coronado began to question the future viability of a small hospital on a small island adjacent to a large city. Through many conversations with their patients and neighbors, the Sharp Coronado team reimagined the entire healthcare experience. Situated on Coronado Island, near the famed Hotel del Coronado, this tiny island gem crafted a new story structure for the physical place by coupling a well-thought-out mini face-lift for the hospital with an extensive design overhaul for every aspect of the patient, employee, and overall hospital experience.

Sharp Coronado Hospital adopted the Planetree philosophy—a set of concepts that focus on humanizing healthcare—and set out to design a place where patients have control over how their care is delivered and where the environment is far more home-like than hospital-like. The team did not have the luxury of creating a brand-new hospital to support their new vision. In fact, they had very little money available to craft a new story structure. But they proved it's possible to succeed in place-making with the right vision, regardless of financial constraints. They created the theme "live+heal+grow" as the cornerstone of their story structure and experience design, and they successfully blended the hospital experience with the larger island experience. The hospital would be a subtle reflection of its island environment—creating a place that would be the most conducive setting for healing and comfort, incorporating nature and a sense of calm. Most San Diegans say that simply driving over the expanse of the Coronado Bay Bridge changes their mind-set and demeanor. So it is with Sharp Coronado Hospital. When you walk through the lobby doors, a feeling of peace and tranquility washes over you.

Capitalizing on the island feel, the team decided to use the subtle island motif of a seashell—but not just any seashell. They selected the nautilus because it is symbolic of an ancient spatial proportioning system, also known as the Fibonacci sequence or the Golden Ratio. It is a ratio that is known to be most pleasing to the human eye and is found throughout nature and across timeless works of art and architecture. So for Sharp Coronado, the nautilus is a symbol of both their island surroundings and the commitment to creating an altogether different and more pleasing healthcare environment and experience.

Now when you walk into the hospital, you see elements of nature and the island. Wood, sand, and water are evoked in the beautiful yet subtle design and décor. The walls are painted in the colors of the sea and the sand. Bamboo, stone, and sea glass serve as harmonizing cues. And wherever possible, curves instead of straight lines are used. And there are no overhead fluorescent lights—lighting is soft and indirect.

Sharp Coronado's "live+heal+grow" theme is also evoked by intentionally bringing the outside in—whether through nature-inspired paint colors or complementary works of art. Garden spaces were transformed into healing spaces and a stunning outdoor labyrinth was recently created to provide a place for mindfulness and reflection.

By using the physical space to serve as the story structure, new roles and behaviors emerge and new stories are created and told. The hospital now has housekeepers dressed in Tommy Bahama–style uniforms, and instead of simply cleaning the rooms, the housekeeping hosts offer warm washcloths twice a day to patients and guests as a special added touch. In the warmer summer months, they provide cool washcloths and lemonade. Volunteer musicians serenade patients and guests, and Traveler, a gorgeous English Sheepdog, provides pet therapy. The hospital is known for baking cookies in the lobby, too.

The hospital offers complimentary therapies to all patients, including clinical aromatherapy, healing touch, and massage. All of the senses were considered in the crafting of the story structure and the new healthcare experience provided to staff members, patients, and guests. The possibilities are endless—even when the budget is not.

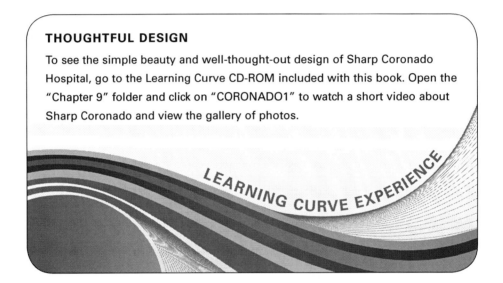

THOUGHTFUL DESIGN

To see the simple beauty and well-thought-out design of Sharp Coronado Hospital, go to the Learning Curve CD-ROM included with this book. Open the "Chapter 9" folder and click on "CORONADO1" to watch a short video about Sharp Coronado and view the gallery of photos.

LEARNING CURVE EXPERIENCE

Art Is Personal

Sharp Memorial Hospital is the flagship facility for the Sharp HealthCare system. The original hospital was envisioned and brought to life more than 50 years ago through the kindness and generosity of the people of San Diego. In the late 1990s, it became obvious that the original hospital would need to expand to meet the ever-changing needs of the community and to comply with California's seismic/

earthquake requirements. So plans were created to build a brand-new Sharp Memorial Hospital adjacent to the original flagship facility. The new Sharp Memorial Hospital would offer all private rooms and unique healing design elements, the latest technology, and thoughtful amenities. The hospital was designed to be extraordinary, and the challenge would be to ensure that a new play would be performed on this glorious stage. How do you create and ensure a new-to-the-world experience and keep old habits, beliefs, and behaviors from walking out the door of the original hospital and into the new one?

For the Sharp Memorial team, it meant using the new structure as the stage for a brand-new performance. The new building sparked the creation of a rich, fresh, well-designed experience. Just three months prior to opening the new hospital, a multidisciplinary team from Sharp Memorial Hospital visited Starizon to immerse themselves in the concepts of experience design and the experience economy. They participated in experience expeditions, learning from some of the best experience stagers. They spent hours defining and designing the New Sharp Memorial Hospital experience.

An operational theme—A Personal Art—was identified to ensure that all decisions regarding the new hospital and new experience fit within the operating theme. A declaration was also created to help define the personal art theme and to help tell the story of what this new hospital would mean to staff members, physicians, patients, and the community.

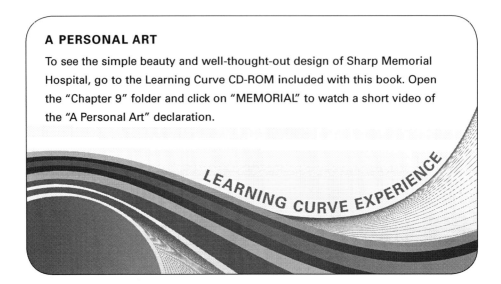

A PERSONAL ART

To see the simple beauty and well-thought-out design of Sharp Memorial Hospital, go to the Learning Curve CD-ROM included with this book. Open the "Chapter 9" folder and click on "MEMORIAL" to watch a short video of the "A Personal Art" declaration.

LEARNING CURVE EXPERIENCE

People Bring the Experience to Life

Although the new hospital, theme, and declaration helped paint a picture of what's possible, the story can be brought to life only by the people who create their daily works of art in that space. To draw the workforce into the new theme and vision, experience ceremonies were held just prior to the planned opening. That was no small feat given that the original hospital was running at capacity and there was just a very small window of time between gaining occupancy of the hospital and the scheduled opening.

Groups of 25 team members at a time were hosted on an interactive experiential tour through the new hospital. Key places within the new facility helped to provide the story structure and punctuate the theme and declaration. There were six stops along the tour, each stop hosted by an experience guide. Meaningful memorabilia was designed and included at each stop along the tour to serve as a poignant reminder of the experience elements that were to be "built in" to the hospital.

The tour started just outside the grand entrance of the hospital with a reminder that the outside of the hospital serves as a symbol of a new future for healthcare, a shining beacon for the community of the limitless possibilities this new hospital brings. Team members were standing (literally) on the threshold of the new hospital, with a blank canvas to create his or her own personal works of art. They were asked to consider their hopes and dreams for the new hospital and to identify the old habits and behaviors they would leave behind.

Once through the doors of the arrival plaza, the first stop was the magnificent Wall of Honor, an artful space honoring the more than 50-year legacy of those who made the hospital possible. It allowed for the legendary stories to be told of the heroes of our organization and served as a reminder that we stand on the shoulders of all those who have come before us, as we continue the vision and quest to create a whole new world of healthcare.

Handcrafted pewter pocket charms were specifically selected to serve as artful memorabilia, coupled with printed quotes that illuminated the key experiential element at each tour stop. A world pocket charm was distributed along with Gandhi's famous quote: "You must be the change you want to see in the world."

The tour proceeded to the Grand Galleria Lobby to share the power and importance of first impressions. One of the hospital's signature moments was shared: a beautiful glass water urn filled with water and fruit. The water urn would provide welcoming refreshment to staff members and guests alike. The acorn pocket charm symbolized warmth and hospitality, and that often, small things can make the biggest difference.

> *The creation of a thousand forests is in one acorn.*
>
> —*Ralph Waldo Emerson*

Guides also shared that bowls of fresh apples would be offered throughout the hospital. The apple represents our commitment to health and vitality and to purposefully bringing the outside in through items from nature.

> *Health is a large word. It embraces not the body only, but the mind and spirit as well; ... and not today's pain or pleasure alone, but the whole being and outlook of a man.*
>
> —*James H. West*

The tours made their way up through the hospital, highlighting the built-in onstage/offstage areas and illuminating the importance of creating a peaceful place for all.

To create a peaceful healing environment for patients and guests, there must be a place of peace and revitalization for staff members as well. The tour included the new staff lounges, honoring team members for the Herculean work they do each day. The lounges would serve as an offstage sanctuary for staff members to refresh and relax, providing them the respite they need to perform their work not as duty, but as art. To ensure that the staff lounges would be personally inspiring, each lounge came equipped with a personalization kit that team members could use to select the inspirational quotes, sayings, and words that would be artfully painted on the walls. The peace sign pocket charm was symbolic of the peace of mind we create for our patients and guests and the peace and balance we create for our staff.

> *The Art of Peace begins with you … foster peace in your own life and then apply the art to all that you encounter.*
>
> —*Morihei Ueshiba*

The next stop was at the heart of the experience: a patient room. This is where the passion of our team members comes to life. It's where we touch the hearts of our patients and where they touch ours. It's where we create a personal art by making their experience as personal as possible—from family sleep beds and personal pajama preferences to custom music and photo offerings. And as much as this is a place of healing, it is also a place of celebration, inspiration, and story.

At the heart of the experience, we will go beyond our patients' medical history to their meaningful story in our attempt to heal the person, not just cure the disease. When we take time to listen, we find the wisdom, wonder, and poetry in the lives and stories of the people we serve. Every single person wants to know that his or her life matters, and when we listen to their stories, we are truly performing an act of love. The heart charm genuinely gets to the heart of the matter.

> *Too often we underestimate the power of a touch, a smile, a kind word, a listening ear, an honest compliment, or the smallest act of caring, all of which have the potential to turn a life around.*
>
> —*Leo Buscaglia*

The highest point in the hospital, with a wall of windows and a beautiful view, was the final stop on the tour. One of the lovely family lounges served as the backdrop for a personal commitment ceremony. It was there that team members were reminded that the height of their accomplishments would equal the depth of their convictions. And that the beauty and majesty of the new building would enhance the artistry and magnificence of the work—work that should be for each and every team member A Personal Art.

The declaration was read aloud and each team member was asked to write and share his or her own personal commitment. There is nothing quite like the beauty and poetry of people's personal commitments.

An angel pocket charm was the final piece of memorabilia presented, and it represented the role that each team member plays as the guardian of the experience we create for each other and for our patients and guests.

> *The greatest achievement was at first and for a time a dream. The oak sleeps in the acorn, the bird waits in the egg, and in the highest vision of the soul a waking angel stirs. Dreams are the seedlings of realities.*
>
> *—James Allen*

At the conclusion of the experience immersion in the new hospital, team members had a better understanding of the part they each play in ensuring that the new hospital structure helped to support a new staff and patient experience that would undoubtedly spark new stories that would soon become legendary.

All these examples illustrate the significant connection that can be made between dramatic structure, story structure, and building structure. When done well, a building is a vibrant training ground that instructs staff members every day on what is intended. And because buildings last for decades, they are a powerful way to communicate to your organization's future leaders, people you will likely never meet, what was believed once upon a time. Winston Churchill had it right when he said, "First we shape our buildings, then they shape us."

THE FAB FOUR:
Make Your Healthcare Organization Legendary

This chapter is not about the British invasion led by four previously unknown chaps from Liverpool who remade music in the 1960s. Rather, it's about the storytelling invasion that will remake the healthcare experience in the next decade, orchestrated by previously unknown operations talent from the marketing department and vibrantly performed by every leader in the organization. With all apologies to the Beatles, "You say you want a revolution, well, you know, there's four roles you gotta play."

Let's look at this new Fab Four and see how they'll change healthcare marketing forever.

The Story Developer

It may seem obvious, but it bears stating: There are no great healthcare stories without great healthcare experiences. That's why progressive marketing departments must take an energetic leap into operations. It is no longer sufficient to chronicle the organization's achievements through creative communications. It is no longer satisfactory to sit outside the executive suite waiting for operating decisions to be made so that you will have something to report. In the experience economy, the experience *is* the marketing, and so marketing professionals must move beyond designing great campaigns to designing great experiences.

It makes all the sense in the world for marketing to play this coordination role, because who better to unify the brand promise with the brand experience than marketers? But although it may be logical, it won't be easy. It will require the development of an operating system no less rigorous than component-based software engineering in IT, generally accepted accounting principles in finance, and comprehensive protocols and care plans in nursing. It will require CEOs to call for their marketing departments to make the transition from communications to operations. It will take professionals in those departments, courageous enough to step well beyond their communications comfort zone, to be the operating change that healthcare so desperately needs. And it will take leaders in every department to be willingly mentored by their marketing counterparts in the new and exciting role of experience producers. Here's how to get started.

Marketing leaders must develop or acquire an experience design and staging operating system. It should be able to be applied to things as big as entire institutions and/or major service lines and as small as signature moments or training classes. It should be broad in its experience philosophy and deep in its implementation modules. And it should, at a minimum, help other operating leaders answer the following six questions:

- What is our organization's theme/storyline and how specifically does my area's experience connect to it?

- How will we make our experience customizable so that it is unique and meaningful at the individual level?

- How will we expand the experience beyond the four walls of our organization to build life-affirming relationships?

- How will we design and prop our physical space to memorably support the experience we are staging?

- How will we inspire patients, families, doctors, and staff members to live our values and work together to carry out a unique brand of healthcare?

- How will we audition, rehearse, award, and critique our work to make sure it becomes "the way" to do things and not a program of the month?

Although these six questions should be a helpful start in your new work as a story developer, they come with a major warning label attached:

> *Warning! Just asking these six questions does not constitute safe and effective use of story development. Developing the systems, processes, and tools needed to consistently answer these questions does.*

Once your story is developed, use of your experience design and staging operating system cannot be optional. It can't be used by some departments and not by others, by some service lines and not by others, by some leaders and not by others. Experiences, like a Broadway play, live and die as a whole. It can't be "piece-mealed" to success. And whether you call them "centers of excellence," "programs of distinction," or "stuff we're really good at," there can be no excellence and distinction without experience excellence and distinction. And it is in the role of the story developer that marketing leaders will ensure that this happens.

The Story Gatherer

One of the biggest reasons that great stories go untold is because they go ungathered. In Chapter 7, we discussed personal stories, including the "Power of One" television spots from Riverside Health System in Newport News, VA. They are powerful tales about how one person can really make a difference.

Every time Gary has shown these spots as an example of great inspirational storytelling in one of his presentations, the audience response is genuine and heartfelt. Every time except one, that is. The group was the senior executive team of a successful healthcare system in the Midwest. They were exploring how experience design and its associated storytelling techniques might help them make a major breakthrough in their already better-than-average performance. After Gary showed the spots, the lights came back up and the healthcare system CEO uttered this amazing insight: "Those stories are really great. I just wish we had some people like that around here."

How do leaders become so isolated from the heart of the work their organizations do, especially in a field such as healthcare? That CEO may know everything about his most profitable diagnosis-related groups, his bond rating, his capital plan, and his key admitting physicians, but he doesn't know anything about the work he

   The Complete Guide to Transforming the Patient Experience

purports to lead. It is an abdication of leadership. And unless it is fixed (which is highly unlikely given his attitude), his healthcare system will never be great.

Not knowing the stories of your organization is a big contribution to the growing divide between managers and employees. Each faction tends to blame the other for the inevitable failings and disappointments all organizations have. Saying, "I wish we had people like that around here" is the same as saying, "This would be a great place if it weren't for the damn employees." And when employees say of their leaders, "They just don't get it," they perpetuate the bungling, sometimes conspiratorial view they have of leaders that is occasionally used to dismiss the attempts even good managers make to improve the place. Stories can bridge this divide, but only if they are gathered in a systematic way and with a particular purpose in mind.

In his book *The Leader's Guide to Storytelling*, Stephen Denning identifies seven distinct purposes a story can serve:

1. Ignite action and spark organizational change
2. Share knowledge
3. Get people working together
4. Lead people into the future
5. Neutralize bad news and gossip
6. Communicate who you are and build trust
7. Transmit values

We highly recommend reading his book for more detail on the specific techniques associated with each purpose. The one point we want to make here is that the whole of the list, the entire seven items taken together, describe something very powerful and very important: the things a great leader does. In fact, if all the leaders in an organization did those seven things, is there any doubt that they and their company would be great? A great leader must be a great storyteller, and you can't be a great storyteller if you are not a great story gatherer.

The first thing marketing leaders have to do in story gathering is set up a system. You won't get close to where you want to go using a haphazard nonmethod, something that is all too common in companies today. Two critical aspects of your story gathering system are establishing story salons and creating story magnets.

Story salons

Story salons are places where people are encouraged to tell the organizational stories they know. A story salon can be held at a department meeting, new employee orientation, a retreat, on rounding, in a performance review, over lunch—almost any setting where the story gatherer consistently elicits and records the company's stories. The more story salons you establish and the more skilled story gatherers you put in them, the bigger story library you'll develop. At Sharp, large group gatherings begin with a story-related icebreaker. Team members pair up and share a story about a recent experience in which they felt most connected and alive in their work, or a story about a recent interaction with a colleague, guest, or patient they feel best exhibited the tenets of The Sharp Experience.

Simply taking the time to get everyone in the room to share a story with a partner, and then report some of the more memorable stories, puts everyone in the role of storyteller and story gatherer. When stories are reported to the group, the twist is that the partner is asked to share the story he or she just heard instead of repeating his or her own story. That helps participants practice, in a safe setting, the act of sharing someone else's story and drawing the entire room into it. Also consider using existing vehicles to support this story gathering process. When you round each day on your staff, choose your words and your questions wisely. Don't simply say, "What's going on?" or "How's everything going?" Say, "Tell me a story about a team member that you are particularly proud of." This can also take place in meetings and when connecting with patients and guests.

Story magnets

Story magnets improve both the quantity and the quality of the stories you gather. The best magnets you have are your established theme and storyline, as well as the organization's mission, vision, and values. These magnets are best used by your ears, not your mouth. In other words, don't say, "Tell me a story about hope, integrity, or exploration." If you direct people in this way, you are likely to hear shallow or contrived tales. It's much better to say, "Tell me a story about someone who works here that really affected you," or "Who inspires you?" Then listen with your theme and storyline, your mission, vision, and values as filters. The story gatherer's contribution is to make the connection in this way and turn interesting personal stories into vibrant corporate ones. Don't be like our forlorn Midwest CEO. There are great stories lying all over the ground at your company. Go out and pick them up.

The Storyteller

Once marketing leaders have made significant progress in story development (through intentional experience design) and story gathering (through establishing story salons and story magnets that other leaders consistently use), you are in great shape to employ all the storytelling techniques we've described throughout this book. Concept stories, personal stories, ceremonial stories, signature moments, rich traditions, and story structures are the new methods of choice. And storytelling is a new way to do things, not just another thing to do. It means much more than just expanding the coverage that stories get in your advertising, newsletters, Web sites, and corporate magazines. It means using stories to run the place—to run the entire company. It is important to remember that the story about what is done is every bit as important as what is actually done. In fact, a great performance that is not embedded in a great story is not a great performance at all because its learning and replication effects are minimized. It will be a great day when most people at your place think you are a great and authentic storytelling company that just happens to be in healthcare, instead of a great healthcare company that just happens to tell stories.

The Story Legendizer

Have you noticed that whether a legendary company has been around for a fairly long time (such as Ogilvy, Nordstrom, Hewlett-Packard, or Apple) or a relatively short time (such as Zappos or Google), it relies on its rich storytelling culture? Maybe that's because legends themselves are a type of story. Now, this is the part where a little concern might be creeping in. You could agree with our premise of

     The Complete Guide to Transforming the Patient Experience

the importance of telling genuine stories in all their forms, but doubt that all your leaders are up to it. They may be reserved or soft spoken. They may be conservative and not into all that "touchy-feely" stuff. There may be lots of problems in your organization right now, so you don't think there are very many good stories to tell. Your executive team may be overwhelmed with all sorts of challenges and you think they don't have time to tell stories. And even if they did, maybe they are the worst after-dinner speakers you have ever heard.

But before you let your inner skeptic take you over, recognize that you must have thought storytelling had some value or you would not have made it this far in the book, and remember that stories aren't just told, they are asked and acted out. Maybe some of your leaders will only be able to ask about and document great stories. After all, the requests to "tell me about something or someone in the company that is who we are when we are at our best" is itself a powerful contribution. Maybe some of your leaders won't say a word, but how and why they do what they do make for an elegant story. Remember, most people would rather see a sermon than hear one any day.

Storytelling and public speaking are not the same thing, so although people may contribute in different ways, they all will be enriched in the same way when storytelling becomes pervasive: Their work and their lives will feel more meaningful when they are surrounded by stories. Corporate folklore helps us remember that we were great and that we will be great again. The stories help us to better understand where we came from, where we are, and where we are going. It is the hope we need in the midst of disappointment. The fun in the midst of struggle. The sparkle in the midst of sameness. The proof in the midst of doubt. There are no great companies that don't have more than their share of recognized great people. And the word *recognized* is just as important as the word *great* in the preceding sentence. It's not enough to simply know that you have great team members doing great work; you must look for the good and choose to recognize it out loud. When a leader tells the story of an individual's achievement out loud and in front of colleagues, the story is imprinted in others and is then far more likely to be replicated.

So recognize great work, reveal it through stories, and repeat it as often as you can. When you legendize storytelling, when you make it an inseparable part of who you are, then you have elevated work from drudgery and duty to discovery and delight. Sometimes, when leaders are within sight of the end of their careers, they wonder what their legacy will be. How will they be remembered? The wise leaders who haven't waited until the end to answer that question realize that the only legacy that matters is the one told today through the stories in their workplace. And the best thing about all those stories is that they will always be remembered.

GETTING REAL:
Close the Gap between Brand Promise and Brand Experience

There's something safe and comforting about those who keep their promises. Think about a person in your life who consistently keeps his or her promises to you. How would you describe that person? Trustworthy? Credible? Honorable? Dependable? Exceptional? Authentic? And what about the opposite kind of person, someone in your life who has a pattern of broken promises? You might call this person unreliable, dishonorable, untrustworthy, insincere, or fake. The same is true for the promises all leaders make, and all too often break, about our brands. We like to think of the brand promise as what we say we are to the outside world. The brand experience is what happens when our patients, guests, and customers actually experience our organizations; it is the reality of who we are.

The Brand Must Be Real

When there is a gap between brand promise and brand experience, our customers question everything about the organization. They become frustrated, lose faith, and tell stories of their own about the perceived and experienced gap between who we say we are and what we really are. These are not the uplifting stories that we've been writing about throughout the book. These are the stories we fear; the stories that are told with or without our knowledge. They are told in face-to-face conversations or they spread like wildfire through the worldwide social media of blogs, YouTube, Facebook, and Twitter. These are the stories that confirm for the world that healthcare (and your organization specifically) will never get better; will never be what people want it to be or what they need it to be. These are the stories that erode confidence, and ultimately erode your organization's brand and the industry's entire reputation.

Marketers work hard to creatively tell the story of the organization (the brand promise) through advertisements, logos, taglines, public relations, magazines, newsletters, events, and more. Our customers expect us not only to deliver on that promise, but also to deliver on it consistently, across the entire organization, with each and every encounter. That takes the commitment of every leader in the place. And when we don't deliver on our promise with the experience we create and stage—even in just one area of our organization or one simple encounter—our customers begin to make broad, sweeping assumptions about who we really are. About our trustworthiness, our credibility, our authenticity. They begin to assume that we must not live the promise anywhere.

How many times have we heard questions such as the following?

     The Complete Guide to Transforming the Patient Experience

If they can't even ...	Then how do I know that they will ...
• Treat me like a human being ...	• Keep me safe?
• Remember my name ...	• Know what they are doing?
• Clean the bathroom ...	• Recommend the right course of action?
• Answer the phone promptly ...	
• Tell me how long it's going to be ...	• Get my medicines right?
• Take my blood on the first try ...	• Perform the surgery on the right body part?
• Make it easy for me ...	
• Anticipate my needs ...	• Take good care of my husband/partner/child/parent/friend?
• Involve my family ...	• Tell me what's happening?
• Remember what's happened in my care so far ...	• Care about my life situation and not just my medical situation?
• Keep me from being exposed to the world in this ridiculous hospital gown ...	• Honor my fears and concerns?

It's a gap that can and will widen exponentially with each broken promise. And it's the reason that so many people think they need an advocate to protect them from the very system that promises to care for them.

If we consider the gap between brand promise and brand experience as a reflection of the gap that too often exists between marketing and operations, or even the gap between the experience we create for our employees and the experience we expect them to create for our customers, the importance of leaders' new roles as story developers, gatherers, tellers, and legendizers comes more clearly into focus.

Maybe some charts and graphs will help us remember this more clearly. In most of healthcare, the brand promise and the brand experience aren't merely two unrelated things; they are worked on by two distinctly different groups of people. Marketing people devote themselves to the promise; operations people devote themselves to the experience. And they don't really see themselves as part of each other's work, as phrases such as "That's a marketing problem, not an operations problem," or vice versa, clearly indicate. These two worlds won't accidentally unite themselves, and the distrust, disappointment, and defection that come from the built-in gap between the two ruin organizations and make greatness impossible.

IS IT REALLY REAL? REALLY?

Inside and outside of healthcare, many marketers are trying to close the gap between marketing and operations using words alone. Look at ads and product packaging over the past couple of years, and you will see an explosion in the use of the words *real, genuine, authentic,* and *original.*

If you go to the Learning Curve CD-ROM included with this book, open the "Chapter 11" folder, and click on "GENUINE," you'll find a sampling of products, services, and experiences that use buzzwords such as *real, genuine, authentic,* and *original.* Isn't it amazing how ubiquitous the terms are, even though it is so rare to truly experience anything that is sincerely real, genuine, authentic, or original?

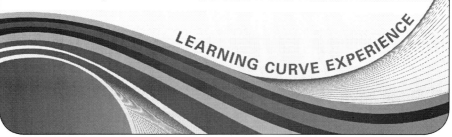

LEARNING CURVE EXPERIENCE

 The Complete Guide to Transforming the Patient Experience

By perpetuating the gap between marketing and operations (see Figure 11.1), we create our own problems.

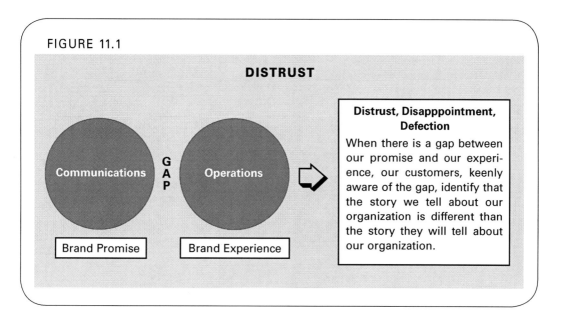

FIGURE 11.1

DISTRUST

Communications

G A P

Operations

Brand Promise

Brand Experience

Distrust, Disapppointment, Defection

When there is a gap between our promise and our experience, our customers, keenly aware of the gap, identify that the story we tell about our organization is different than the story they will tell about our organization.

Joe Pine and Jim Gilmore, in their latest book *Authenticity—What Consumers Really Want*, put it well:

> *No matter what the nature of the offerings you sell, stop fretting about the declining efficacy of advertisements and pay more attention to how the ads represent those offerings to your current and potential customers. Companies so often behave in ways that render their own offerings inauthentic. By word or deed—via marketing activities or designed offerings—businesses all too often produce their own fakes.*

Healthcare is too important to fake, so not only must we stop conceiving of communications, operations, promise, and experience as separate things, but also we must start intentionally bringing them together. (See Figure 11.2.)

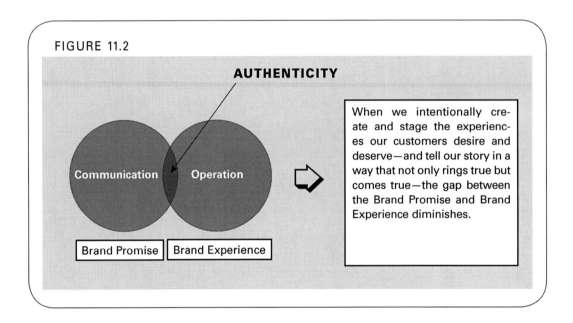

FIGURE 11.2

AUTHENTICITY

Communication   Operation

Brand Promise   Brand Experience

When we intentionally create and stage the experiences our customers desire and deserve—and tell our story in a way that not only rings true but comes true—the gap between the Brand Promise and Brand Experience diminishes.

The greater the area of overlap, the more authenticity and brand power we are creating. The closer we get to concentric circles, the more delight, desire, and devotion we will see from our customers. And the more they will help us do our jobs. (See Figure 11.3.)

    The Complete Guide to Transforming the Patient Experience

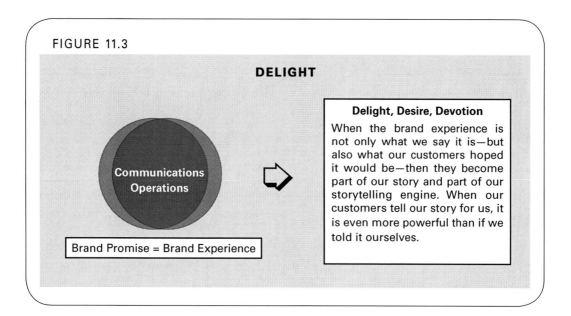

FIGURE 11.3

DELIGHT

Communications
Operations

Brand Promise = Brand Experience

Delight, Desire, Devotion

When the brand experience is not only what we say it is—but also what our customers hoped it would be—then they become part of our story and part of our storytelling engine. When our customers tell our story for us, it is even more powerful than if we told it ourselves.

In Chapter 3, we asked you to consider the notion put forward in Pine and Gilmore's "Experience IS the Marketing" whitepaper that "people have become relatively immune to messages targeted at them. The way to reach your customers is to create experiences within them." As such, we believe that all marketing really begins at the bedside—in places and spaces where our patients, guests, and customers interact with our team members. It is there in patient and procedure rooms, at the concierge and in the cafeteria, on the phone or online. When our people bring the best of who they are to our patients, they create experiences for them, with them, and ultimately within them.

You Have to Be Real

To create and render authentic, positively memorable healthcare experiences for patients—and help change their story—we must begin by focusing on our employees and their "work story."

As we shared in Chapter 4, our ability to succeed in the experience economy requires us to create the best experience for our team members so that they can create the best experience for our patients and customers. So it is with rendering authenticity in this work. All leaders must be real for and with their team members so that team members can be real, and really great, for and with customers. Otherwise, team members will see right through insincere attempts to make the experience better. To avoid this, leaders must be real in 12 specific ways.

1. Real as visionaries

Leaders must be real in their vision and intention. Does the vision paint a clear picture of a brighter future in a way that team members can believe and rally behind? Do the leaders "act as if" the vision has already been achieved in how they decide things on a daily basis? And do they go first in this commitment despite what other leaders may do or the budget may say?

2. Real as people

Leaders must be real in who they are to team members. Every move we make and every word we speak is onstage for our team members to observe and assess—to create their own judgments about how genuine we are. Do we truly walk the talk? Are we role models for exactly what we want and expect our team members to live?

 The Complete Guide to Transforming the Patient Experience

3. Real in standards, expectations, and accountability

As a leadership team, do we hold ourselves accountable in the same way we hold team members accountable, or do we create a special class of privilege and exception to govern our actions?

4. Real in the relationships they nurture

Our team members want to believe that we really want to know them and that we have what it takes to care for and about them. Nurturing relationships with our team members is not a once-in-a-lifetime activity. It is a daily commitment. Nurturing relationships puts the focus on the person—not the profession.

5. Real in their understanding of who they serve

Team members like to connect with experiences that tie to their innate sense of self. If the experience is something that really connects to who they are as people, they are more likely to value it and more likely to confirm the idea by saying, "I like that. I'm like that." Team members not only demand experiences, but demand for them to be real and meaningful to them on an individual basis.

6. Real in the stories they tell

Whether in personal, context, or spatial stories, leaders must tell the real story of where we've been, where we are, and where we're going. Authentic stories build trust, and for workers in healthcare, trust is required.

7. Real in the manner in which they gather stories

The stories leaders choose to tell must come from the organic, original elements of the work. They can't be fabricated or fictional.

8. Real in the information they share

Increased transparency and public reporting hold our organizations to that which is real—shining a light on the real outcomes, the real experience. It also requires leaders to get real in their willingness to hold up the organizational mirror and not pretend to see beauty when the image is scary and ugly.

9. Real in who they recognize and legendize

When we choose to hold up someone as a legend, an example, and as the new standard, we must ensure that he or she is the real deal. That this person indeed lives the vision, standards, and experience. If leaders don't do their due diligence—and they hold up low or inconsistent performers for political reasons—high performers will be turned off immediately.

10. Real in the desire to listen, to learn, and to change

Creating a new experience in healthcare is difficult. It takes hard work and perseverance. And it takes thick skin. Leaders have to really want to listen, to learn from what they hear and change their organizations and, more importantly, change themselves as a result.

11. Real in their desire to make the healthcare experience better

They must be committed to making the healthcare experience everywhere, not just inside their own organization and not just for their organization's own financial rewards. If leaders are not genuinely committed—in word and deed—to transforming the healthcare experience for everyone, they won't successfully engage their team members in anything more than a charade.

These 11 items may seem like an incredible amount of work. You might think you can't possibly do and be all of those things. But before you close this book and try something else that seems more attainable, we'd like to suggest a 12th way of being real that makes the other 11 a little less daunting:

12. Real about mistakes

You will not always do the right thing, at the right time, in the right way. You just won't. And being real about the mistakes you make by openly admitting them, expressing sadness about falling short of your own aspirations, and promising to try again in a wiser way will endear you to the people you lead. It will also break you out of what we like to call "perfection prison." That's the place where skeptics, cynics, and bystanders, at all levels in an organization, trap people who are committed to possibility and transformation. It usually sounds something like this: "How do I know this isn't just another program of the month? I think I'll wait and see." Or "I've seen these change programs come and go along with the leaders that started them. I'm still here and they're not." Or "I want to see whether they are really committed and that this experience thing really works before I get on board." Or "I know most of the leaders are trying to do it, but several are really resisting. So what's the point?" Or "My boss says and does a lot of the right things to make this change, but every now and then, he reverts to his old ways. I can't trust him." And the "Perfection Prison Blues" goes on and on and on. No matter how the verses change, the chorus is always the same: "Until my leaders are perfect in their dedication and their actions, I don't have to do anything."

This kind of attitude can paralyze the best of organizations, even if it's held by only a relatively small amount of people. As Peter Block discusses in his book

Stewardship: Choosing Service over Self Interest, leaders enable this power precisely by not admitting their mistakes, expressing disappointment in themselves, and trying again to do better. Hiding mistakes gives them power. Admitting them and doing better gives you power. You are essentially saying, "I am choosing this new and difficult path in spite of the failures of the past, both mine and the company's. It is important to the success of the company and my personal beliefs. I am inviting you to make the same choice." As a leader, there is no mistake that you can't ultimately recover from, other than the mistake of not admitting your mistakes and promising to do better next time. How you handle mistakes can make you more real than how you handle success.

The experiences we create and stage at the bedside, however elaborate or simple, generate the stories our patients will tell about our organizations. The experiences we create and stage in meetings big or small generate stories our team will tell about us as leaders. These two sets of stories will determine whether we are perceived as real, genuine, and authentic or as untrustworthy, unreliable, and fake. This perception is every bit as important in your work life as it is in your personal life. We are imploring you, no matter what area you lead, to take on new roles and responsibilities that blur the lines between marketing and operations. We are pleading with you to flip the traditional model of marketing from one that starts with the brand promise and hopes for a worthy brand experience, to one that starts with the rich and comprehensive crafting of the brand experience in a way that creates a brand promise that you can share with authenticity and meaning.

Because, after all, the promise matters only if we live it.

A NOTE FROM THE AUTHORS

The World of the Asterisk

I'm sure you've never had the occasion to ponder all the meanings and uses of that tiny piece of punctuation called the asterisk. Sonia and I hadn't, either, until we decided to add it to the title of our book and use to inspire the cover design as well. I guess we knew that, by definition, the asterisk is intended to call attention to something, highlight something special, or show something interesting or important. When we added it to the word "complete" in our title, we wanted to make sure that everyone knew, right away, how important and essential your contribution of talent, passion, and hard work is. Without it, none of what we've learned about and written about experience design and staging really matters. It would never be "complete."

We also like that the word asterisk contains the word "risk," because you will definitely be taking some when you follow our advice. As you know, risk is a requirement of any breakthrough. The root words of asterisk mean "little star" and those willing to take actions as a result of this book will be just that—they will illuminate the new path healthcare so desperately needs.

It is also cool that in math the asterisk indicates multiplication—because the personal aspect of experience work is the ultimate multiplier—creating even greater outcomes through personal passion than could ever be achieved by simply following a written prescription.

Sonia has some computer programming in her background and she informed me that the asterisk was used as a wild card. In the old DOS days, *.* indicated "ALL Files." Our asterisk is also a wild card that means "all." If you bring all of your talent, all of your passion, and all of your hard work, you will get all of the results you are looking for.

All of these meanings, however, would have remained a kind of authors' "secret code" had something extraordinary not happened to me shortly before this book went to print. Sonia and I were at the 2009 Pine and Gilmore thinkAbout in Philadelphia. In retrospect, given the huge impact over the years that thinkAbout has made in our lives, our work, and our friendship, it's not surprising that it held a magnificent, if last-minute, additional insight for our book.

I was waiting for the opening session to begin and introducing myself to the participants around me when Sonia excitedly brought me an article from that morning's *USA Today* entitled, "The World of Asterisk."

 The Complete Guide to Transforming the Patient Experience

When you work on something as long and hard as we have on this book, you are constantly looking for signs that you're on the right path. The timing of this little gift from the universe couldn't have been better. It's what happened next, however, that was the truly remarkable part.

The article was about expanding the use of the asterisk from the world of tainted sports records, such as the number of Barry Bonds' home runs, to other fields of endeavor such as politics, business, and journalism, where some famous and influential people have acted in a way far removed from real and genuine. It's an interesting idea, but the real insight came from a man who just happened to be seated next to me. After briefly scanning the article, he offered this gem: "You know, the asterisk is a not-so-silent plea for authenticity." A not-so-silent plea for authenticity—you could have knocked me out of my chair with a feather. That's exactly what it is and the most important reason there is no better symbol for this book and for your work.

Authenticity through the fulfilling of a creative brand promise through an intentional brand experience. Authenticity in the words and actions of healthcare leaders. And authenticity from passionate work that unites the head and the heart. This is our not-so-silent plea to you.

Thanks for listening.

Gary Adamson

What's Your Story?

The methods, examples, and stories you've read about in this book are all genuine and true. (They'd better be, considering what we wrote about authenticity in the preceding chapter.) They have been tried and tested by me (and my 14,000 team-mates) at Sharp HealthCare and by my coauthor, Gary Adamson, in companies in and out of healthcare all across the country. They have led to our organization's success and national recognition—Sharp's National Malcolm Baldrige Award and Starizon's designation by Inc. magazine as one of the 500 fastest growing, private-ly held companies. Gary and I were the cowinners of Pine & Gilmore's first Experience Management Award and have had the opportunity to share our story and our success with thousands of people at national conferences and public forums. It's all been very gratifying and humbling for both of us.

But that's not the real story or the main reason we hope you put our insights to work at your organization. The ultimate reason is what doing and living this work has meant to Gary and me. And what it can mean to you. We've had the chance to elevate our practice of leadership and, to some degree, the respect and expectations of people throughout the healthcare field.

We've seen the tear-streaked faces of healthcare professionals as they express the joy of finding the lost meaning of their work and achieving the purpose they had when they decided to go into healthcare in the first place. We have been a part of attempts to do the "impossible" that have succeeded beyond anyone's wildest imagination.

We have felt the personal satisfaction that comes from changing a small part of the world and a large part of ourselves. But most of all, we have started to change the story of what healthcare could be and, more importantly, will be. We've at least written the prelude, through our work, of the healthcare that we want for our parents, our children, and ourselves. We have written down everything we've learned, our entire learning curve—our complete* guide.

Our experience means you can use it as a confident starting point in your work. And although this is the end of our book, it is just the beginning of your story. What story will you write through your deeds? Make it a bestseller.

Here's to creating positively memorable healthcare experiences.

Sonia Rhodes

FREE HEALTHCARE COMPLIANCE AND MANAGEMENT RESOURCES!

Need to control expenses yet stay current with critical issues?

Get timely help with FREE e-mail newsletters from HCPro, Inc., the leader in healthcare compliance education. Offering numerous free electronic publications covering a wide variety of essential topics, you'll find just the right e-newsletter to help you stay current, informed, and effective. All you have to do is sign up!

With your FREE subscriptions, you'll also receive the following:

- Timely information, to be read when convenient with your schedule
- Expert analysis you can count on
- Focused and relevant commentary
- Tips to make your daily tasks easier

And here's the best part—there's no further obligation— just a complimentary resource to help you get through your daily challenges.

It's easy. Visit *www.hcmarketplace.com/free/e-newsletters* to register for as many free e-newsletters as you'd like, and let us do the rest.

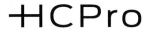 HCPro | Insight for healthcare compliance and management